CONTENTS

<u>P.S.</u>
<u>The Ultimate Miriam Makeba Playlist</u>

DEDICATION

For Caroline McDonald, Anita van de Wetering and Paul Hokkeling, three great Dutmella Scouting friends who passed away when we were teens. To Barry van Loon, my best friend's brother, to Rita Geven, my dear friend John's sister, and to my beloved uncle Nico, dad's younger brother. Meredith Somers, you are missed dearly.

Forever young, never forgotten.

Adhesive arachnoiditis is the absolute abyss of existence, a complete and utter annihilation of what it means to be human. And yet, within that emptiness, that bleakness, I found humanity in myself, and most importantly, in others. - K.G.

"There is mounting evidence that for both the acutely suicidal and those suffering from chronic depression [and/or pain-K.G.], time lost is brain lost is lives lost. Finding more rapidly acting and more effective therapies is essential." - Stephen J. Hyde, M.D., The Ketamine Papers[1]

DEFINITIONS

Cauda equina syndrome = damage to the bundle of nerves below the end of the spinal cord, aka CES.

Causalgia = a constant, usually burning pain that results from injury to a peripheral nerve: e.g., complex regional pain syndrome, or CRPS.

Neuralgia = intense, typically intermittent pain along the course of a nerve: e.g., trigeminal neuralgia, post-herpetic neuralgia (pain after shingles).

Neuroinflammatory = inflammation of nervous tissue aka neuritis.

Neurological = anatomy, functions, and disorders of nerves and nervous system.

Neuropathic pain = pain generated by nerve damage or disease; if caused by brain or spinal cord lesion it's referred to as *central* neuropathic pain syndrome.

Neuropathy = disease or dysfunction of one or more peripheral nerves, typically causing numbness or weakness: e.g., diabetic neuropathy, carpal tunnel syndrome, small fiber neuropathy.

Adhesive arachnoiditis = thickening and adhesions of the leptomeninges in the brain or spinal cord, resulting from previous *meningitis*, or other disease process or trauma; it is sometimes secondary to therapeutic or diagnostic injection of substances into the subarachnoid space. The signs and symptoms vary with extent and location. - Dorland's Medical Dictionary.

INTRODUCTION

Out of desperation, we started providing ketamine infusions. There was nothing left we could offer our patients. - Rio Grande Hospital Pain Management Team

By the end of 2015, the physical agony and suffering had become so pervasive, I started yet another Google document titled "My Suicidal Year." I was done with this body, and this life, but gave myself twelve more months to turn things around, while searching for relief. Ketamine had long been on my mind as a possible treatment; between January and June of 2017, I had nine outpatient ketamine infusions, followed by a weeklong in-patient ketamine treatment. It dampened the soul-sucking pain and may have halted the 'meningeal' inflammation—the lining that covers your brain, central nervous system and spinal cord roots.

Since ketamine infusions, I've noticed a significant change in pain. My body feels as if it belongs to me again, despite profound neurological and musculoskeletal damage—nerve, bone and joint problems. Ketamine's side-effects may deter some, a quiet room, dimmed lights, relaxing music and sedating medication can make a difference. Even with those aides, I had such vivid dreams and sensations it scared me. The pain relief was immediate though, and over the years, I learned to lose that fear. My focus is on the physical healing and transformational aspect of ketamine; even the PTSD from the sky diving accident has much improved.

As an author-patient I won't just invite you into my world, I'm fully transparent. Most books, no matter how wonderful, do not disclose the author's medications and dosages, whereas I think it's helpful to explain what pharmaceuticals are needed, for someone with grave neuropathic pain. Spoiler alert: at the end of this book I am still disabled—ketamine won't miraculously heal decades old crushed sacral nerves—*and* I still live alone. Many beautiful books and uplifting memoirs have been published by writers who conquered their disease and/or transcended their physical circumstances.

Some inspiring authors regained a fully functioning life, others are married or partnered, with seemingly a tad more physical, social and/or financial support. I'm in the States, 5147 miles away from my family, and this is my story. However, I'm far from alone: although most of my anguish is caused by 'cauda equina syndrome' and 'adhesive arachnoiditis,' around 40 million Americans suffer from neuropathic pain, an astounding 10-12.5% of the population.[2]

* * *

I refer to the past in order to illustrate the present, but *The Queen of Ketamine* mostly deals with events from August 2015 through September 2017. It morphed into an evidence-based memoir, and practical guide; though for every chapter that is heavy on medical terminology you will find lighthearted ones such as "Be Careful of the K-Hole, Yo!"

Read this book as you see fit: the Introduction focuses on ketamine and its properties, Part One contains an in-depth chapter on the nighttime skydiving accident, followed by a chapter on my youth, moving from Detroit to Socorro, and the unfortunate lumbar puncture which may have led to neuroinflammation. Part Two is on the physical hell of neuropathic pain and its multiple causes, becoming bedridden and more desperate, yet still wanting to date. Let's just say I was *extremely* motivated to get laid at least once, before I die.

"Welcome to Hell," chapter 4, contains the most clinical terms, medical explanations and background. Part Three is filled with ketamine infusion adventures, stand-up comedy, my perennial pitfalls and an Afterword. Part Four features pragmatic tips for living with any chronic physical and/or psychiatric disorder, stem cell pros and cons, ketamine prescription examples and more. This book ends with Resources, a P.S., Acknowledgments, Miriam Makeba playlist and footnotes.

Ketamine clinics, useful websites and "Kaatje's Favorite Things" can be found in the Resources section. My Amazon public wish list has the books mentioned, practical, stylish home modifications and back pain tools. Think of "Kaatje's Favorite Things" as a benevolent and much more affordable Oprah, or GOOP, shopping guide, where instead of spending $600 for an organic cashmere sweater, you'll own 10 great books, and 14-16 handy medical items, for $580.[3] Take that, Oprah and Gwyneth!

* * *

If you're a medical provider reading this book, whether as a MD, NP, PA, nurse, OT, PT, psychologist, caregiver or other: kudos, you will understand neuropathic pain and treatment better than most of your colleagues. You've probably already encountered patients with 'adhesive arachnoiditis,' an underdiagnosed, progressive *neuroinflammatory* disorder of the meningeal layer. You couldn't have known, for the medical file may state 'radiculopathy' or 'Failed Back Surgery Syndrome.'

Professional medical education at any level—even physicians who specialize in Radiology—aren't taught the signs or symptoms of adhesive arachnoiditis, or back pain with a neuropathic component. And occasionally, it *is* hard to visualize, since adhesions may be present in hidden spots. This is why Primary Care providers will make the biggest difference in the neuropathic pain epidemic: by carefully listening to patients' complaints pointing to neurological involvement, then provide support and appropriate treatment. (With or without an MRI showing abnormalities.)

And why are Primary Care providers our greatest hope for diagnosing and managing neuropathic pain? There simply aren't enough Pain Medicine specialists to cope with the 12.5% of population suffering from neuropathy, and/ or adhesive arachnoiditis. When I use the term adhesive arachnoiditis, this concerns the chronic form, since some patients may have acute arachnoiditis and recover. Be alert when you hear, or have, complaints such as *burning*, *gnawing* or *electrical sensations*, and the inability to sit or stand without excruciating pain. Adhesive arachnoiditis, central pain syndrome (e.g., post-stroke, multiple sclerosis, Parkinson's), trigeminal neuralgia, CRPS (chronic regional pain syndrome), alcoholism, cluster headaches, Ehlers-Danlos syndrome, diabetic neuropathy, fibromyalgia, post-cancer neuropathies, phantom limb pain, cauda equina syndrome (CES) and others may all cause severe, neuropathic pain.

Words such as *intractable* and *incurable* bring an extra dimension to an underestimated, enormous public health issue. Pain that is *extremely hard to treat* and cannot be cured leads to an individual and societal burden of epic proportions, not just physical but in a financial sense too. It requires multi-modal treatment such as ketamine infusions, anti-seizure medications, opioids, at home Toradol injections, intermittent steroids, hospitalizations and rehabilitation. Scientists, researchers and medical providers argue that intractable pain ought to be recognized as its own disorder: ICD 10 code R52.10 allows providers reimbursement for *chronic intractable pain* treatment and diagnosis.

The suffering of adhesive arachnoiditis has been compared to that of metastatic, terminal cancer, according to the National Organization for Rare Diseases.[4] And yes, I've got a stand-up joke about that. Very few physicians specialize in treating and diagnosing adhesive arachnoiditis. Dr. Antonio Aldrete correctly identified that many patients with 'Failed Back Surgery Syndrome' suffer from adhesive arachnoiditis, his article "Suspecting and Diagnosing Adhesive Arachnoiditis" remains a classic.[5]

Dr. Burton has an extensive website which includes the Derek Morrison hypothesis that President JFK suffered from lumbosacral adhesive arachnoiditis, after injection with Pantopaque® caused chemical meningitis. [6], [7] Prominent Pain Medicine specialist Dr. Forest Tennant has treated intractable pain since 1975, he publishes articles, books and neuroinflammatory protocols for adhesive arachnoiditis and Ehlers-Danlos syndrome.[8] I remain a tad skeptical that overdosing on turmeric is beneficial, although his advice on neurohormones, daily stretching and exercise will help you survive. With or without a pain disorder, the human body is meant to move, whether actively or passively.

* * *

Let me emphasize that my personal experience with ketamine's unique pain relief properties should not be used as testimony. We must rely on statistics; my positive response cannot be applied to everyone who suffers from neuropathic agony, or a psychiatric disorder. Remember: correlation is not causation. But ketamine treatment is worth trying, and best of all, it is non-invasive.

When I refer to ketamine this is 'Ketalar' medication, a so-called 'racemic' mixture, with both S- and R-stereoisomer structure. The patented, expensive *esketamine* intranasal spray that came on the market in 2019 has an S-enantiomer structure only. Ketamine infusions (IV) do not work for all patients. Still, I urge you not to give up. Some patients respond better to oral, intramuscular (IM) injection or intranasal ketamine than IV. It may be that lower doses work better, sometimes higher doses, regardless of delivery mode.

I consider myself lucky: my body immediately responds to the infusions. As soon as the ketamine IV is running it feels like a cold, soothing shower deep inside my body. (Instead of feeling as if molten lead is poured from waist to legs.) To my delight, after a ketamine infusion, it seems my brain has access to wonder again—my default setting. From enjoying a beautiful day to quicker connections in my mind, I even recall memories more vividly. In combination with a body that functions better, this is no minor miracle. That said, I fully acknowledge, whether as a patient or provider, you may not have access to ketamine infusions or medication.

You might live in a rural area too far away from a clinic, or your health insurance doesn't approve treatment, and you cannot afford an infusion. Even so, this memoir will motivate you to keep going, to transcend feelings of isolation and gut-wrenching ache. Incorporate self-care and stretching; learn tools to help manage your chronic illness. Show your Primary Care provider, or your Pain Management team, how to prescribe oral or intranasal ketamine, which can be mailed to you from a compounding pharmacy—see Ketamine at Home, under Resources. Don't give up hope, even without access to ketamine. Things will change.

In 2018, much-needed Ketamine Consensus Guidelines for acute and chronic pain conditions were published, this is a great source for patients and providers.[9] Another article, "Intravenous Ketamine Infusions for Neuropathic Pain Management: A Promising Therapy in Need of Optimization" explains: "[…] ketamine infusions have been studied in the treatment of complex regional pain syndrome (CRPS), spinal cord injury, phantom limb pain, postherpetic neuralgia, fibromyalgia, and oncologically mediated neuropathic pain. Additional prospective studies also suggest a role for ketamine infusion therapy in the treatment of trigeminal neuropathic pain, acute and chronic migraines, and temporomandibular pain."[10] It's not that hard to read for non-scientists, and as a patient, it helps being informed. Just make sure that whatever you read comes from a reputable source, such as NIH, PubMed or Google Scholar.

* * *

The fact is that most patients need frequent maintenance infusions, a few will not respond to IV ketamine and a small number gets by with yearly infusions. No one doubts however that ketamine is radically changing patients' lives. Jonathan DelosSantos, PA-C and Clinical Administrator for Ketamine Wellness Centers, via personal communication: "For CRPS and fibromyalgia the success rate is about 85% - 90%. For migraine headaches it's about a 50% response rate. For depression it's about 80% and depression with anxiety, about 75%. For statistical purposes, the success rate is based on the percent reduction in either the pain index or depression index, depending on the condition being treated."

Jonathan adds: "The majority of responders need a maintenance schedule. It is unfortunately rare for patients to stabilize and not need another treatment for another one to two years, perhaps as little as 1 to 2 percent of patients." Dr Theodore Henderson, in a psychiatric setting, observes a response of 80-85% by using a slightly different, and perhaps somewhat more affordable, protocol: averaging 4.3 infusions over 5-7 weeks instead of three infusions a week for two weeks. (Oral antidepressants on the other hand, have a 42-59% response rate after 12 weeks, according to British research.)[11] Dr Henderson postulates that although ketamine provokes an immediate anti-suicidal effect, neuroplasticity and brain repair take a few weeks to develop after an infusion, so there may be no need to administer multiple infusions at the onset.[12]

Additionally, ketamine appears to have profound neuroregenerative and anti-inflammatory properties; it seems bowel and bladder functioning, joint aches and skin sensation have all improved. The soles of my feet, the back of my legs and buttocks remain numb, but my left ankle sensation has normalized somewhat. Medical providers attribute these results to *normal* nerve signals surfacing, instead of the neuropathic torment hijacking my spinal cord and brain. But ketamine and I know better: there's something special about compound CI-581.

* * *

The journey of ketamine began with the brilliant work of Professor Stevens in Detroit. In 1962, as a Parke Davis Consultant and Organic Chemistry professor at Wayne State University, Calvin Stevens synthesized a compound similar to phencyclidine, but without its prolonged, severe side effects. Ketamine's exceptional story continued with University of Michigan Professors Domino (Pharmacology) and Corssen (Anesthesiology).[13]

They first administered the new anesthetic to human volunteers in 1964, ran a small trial in 1965 and by 1966 found that over 130 surgical patients tolerated ketamine well, from age six weeks to 86 years. Their 1965 research paper, "Pharmacologic effects of CI-581, a new dissociative anesthetic, in man" is a great read. Their observation "[...] *this drug is an effective analgesic and anesthetic agent in doses of 1.0 to 2.0 mg. per kilogram*" is especially poignant: the 2018 Consensus Guidelines recommends a 0.5-2 mg per kilogram dose, for chronic pain.[14] By 1970 ketamine was approved by the FDA. Professor Domino's wife Toni came up with the moniker "dissociative anesthetic."[15]

No one, medical providers nor fellow patients, and definitely not the media, can fully prepare you for ketamine's dissociative effects though. They are intensely personal experiences that may seem completely at odds with how you have known your world, and even your own *self* for decades. This is what drugs.com, a reputable website, states about ketamine's side-effects: "Holding false beliefs that cannot be changed by fact, blurry vision, seeing, hearing, or feeling things that are not there, confusion as to time, place, or person, dream-like state." Nope. That is not what ketamine feels, like to me.

Additionally, I would explain to patients: *you might feel as if there is no 'you', your mind will take you inside an elevator all the way up to the Universe, an excellent vantage point from where you'll witness, feel and experience civilizations rise and fall, a thousand times over, you observe Planet Earth covered with the skeletons of humanity's ancestors yet it won't be frightening. You may feel like you're flying for hours in a different dimension, you will try to pee mid-treatment, but your legs look as if they no longer belong to your body. And sometimes you'll feel as if you are locked up in a box. Most importantly though, if you are lucky, your suffering will be greatly lessened, your psyche transformed, and side effects stop quickly after the infusion is stopped.*

* * *

Should you be concerned that racemic ketamine is not FDA approved, except for the pricey intranasal spray, Spravato? Dr Theodore Henderson, in his *Psychiatry Advisor* article, states: "What most Americans do not know is that FDA approval simply means that a company has government permission to advertise the drug for a specific disease. For example, aspirin is used to treat headaches, prevent strokes, prevent heart attacks, relieve pain, treat arthritis, and reduce fever; however, it is *only* approved by the FDA for fever and pain relief. So, utilizing ketamine for depression is no different from using aspirin to prevent strokes and heart attacks."[16]

What about ketamine abuse, addiction or dependence? Drug addiction centers, and most media, seem to push a harmful and sensationalist narrative. By demonizing and spreading lies about ketamine, the addiction treatment clinics benefit financially. According to drugabuse.com, a portal for

American Addiction Centers: "Ketamine was originally developed as an alternative to PCP, but it had *more* powerful side effects, so it was relegated to animals."[17] Uh, no. Sure, ketamine was synthesized as an alternative to phencyclidine (PCP) but quickly gained medical acceptance because the side effects are *less* powerful, roughly 1/10 of PCP's.[18]

Even the Surgeon General's website erroneously states ketamine causes respiratory depression.[19] If it does hamper breathing, that most likely means other drugs were present, like heroin, benzodiazepines, fentanyl or alcohol, all of which depress breathing and increase the risks of aspiration. Ketamine is the go-to surgical anesthetic in developing nations, without an anesthesiologist or electricity, since it does *not* depress breathing.

Taking illicit ketamine is dangerous because a user won't know its quality, and other toxins or drugs may be present. This is why the Netherlands has a harm reduction strategy: users may bring their very small, personal supply, such as meth, MDMA, ketamine, cocaine, LSD etc., to an addiction clinic for purity testing. The trained provider testing the substances also explains the user how to reduce risks like overdose, hyperthermia and dehydration.[20]

The reality is that a small percentage of humans will use drugs recreationally and habitually, yet many users will try illicit drugs for a limited period of time and move on. In an illegal setting, much higher doses of ketamine—and contaminants—will be used than what is provided to an in- or outpatient, which can cause severe bladder disease. However, the most abused, and the deadliest substances in the US are nicotine and alcohol.[21]

* * *

Dutch statistics from 2013 show that 97.9% of all nicotine, alcohol and drug deaths were caused by alcohol and nicotine (21,513 total), and 2.1% (99 total) from illegal drugs.[22] Compare that with the USA, where 88.75 % of all nicotine, alcohol and drug annual deaths were due to alcohol and nicotine (568,000 total) and 11.25% (72,000) from drugs, or rather, *mixed use overdose* deaths, illicit fentanyl being the main culprit in 2017.[23]

These numbers indicate that in the US, alcohol and nicotine annually kill 0.18% of the population, whereas "only" 0.13% of the Dutch will die—this 0.05% difference is not statistically significant. Where the numbers most shockingly diverge is annual, mixed use overdose deaths: 0.022% of the US population will die, vs 0.00062% of the Dutch.[24] In North-America, two trends have emerged regarding recreational ketamine use: first, if ketamine was present in ER visits, in 71.5% of cases alcohol was the other abused drug, and secondly, ketamine use has decreased in age 12 and up.[25]

One of the Rio Grande Hospital attending physicians states, via personal communication: "Ketamine is used post-surgery for patients with heroin or opioid use disorder, it provides those patients pain control and seems to lessen cravings for illicit drug use." The WHO comments, in its fact file on ketamine: "Worldwide, ketamine misuse occurs on a relatively small scale, and PCP derivatives constituted only 1% of 'new psychoactive substances,'" according to the UN Office of Drugs and Crime.[26]

Sadly, the media hardly ever broadcasts this viewpoint: "The WHO Committee concluded that ketamine abuse does *not* pose a global public health threat, while controlling it could limit access to the only anaesthetic and pain killer available in large areas of the developing world."[27] *Discover* magazine is one of the few mainstream publications that gets it right: "From Popular Anesthetic to Antidepressant, Ketamine Isn't the Drug You Think It Is."[28]

Even my beloved *Scientific American* stated: "Is the Ketamine Boom Getting out of Hand? The anesthetic and *party drug* offer depression patients new hope, but some clinics may stray from science."[29] Duh. *Wired*: "Patients Are Experimenting With Ketamine to Treat Depression. Dozens of clinics across the nation are using ketamine—*also known as the club drug Special K*—to treat depression."[30] First, why use a tired cliché, instead of *also known as an essential, lifesaving medication?*

Secondly, ought we not consider that people with depression are predisposed to experiment with MDMA and ketamine, precisely *because* they have failed multiple SSRIs and SNRIs? Ok *Wired*, what else do you got: "Ketamine Stirs Up Hope—and Controversy—as a Depression Drug."[31] Meh. A few paragraphs into the otherwise must-read article, the off-label use pops up without an adequate explanation, and of course, the ubiquitous club drug reference, without statistics.

Is it any wonder that my own mother, upon learning I was writing this book, worryingly said: "But sweetheart, isn't ketamine dangerous, and really addictive?"

"Mom, your precious first born is alive because of ketamine!"

* * *

After reading *The Ketamine Papers* and *Ketamine for Depression* I quickly realized that access to—oral—ketamine treatment ought to be a major goal for the UN, WHO and The Melinda and Bill Gates Foundation. Ketamine certainly will decrease the sheer number of lives lost to suicide—one million a year, globally—yet it is useful for so much that ails humanity. Ketamine is used for obsessive compulsive disorder, alcohol and drug use disorders, PTSD, anxiety, eating and mood disorders. Case reports even show a positive response for schizophrenia, priapism, asthma, epilepsy, bipolar disease and excited delirium.[32]

Ketamine must be tried sooner, not just for the management of chronic pain, but also as palliative care medicine and for end-of-life anxiety. The magnitude of suffering cannot be underestimated; people with schizophrenia, bipolar disorder and treatment resistant depression, on average, die 20 years earlier compared to their non-affected peers.[33] As a Paramedic in training, we took a field trip to University of Michigan Hospital's burn center. Ketamine is so useful in those settings, it seems criminal to withhold this versatile, safe medication during the agony of skin debridement, or for minor emergencies and procedures.[34]

India has successfully trained peer psychiatric workers because the need to treat mental health is so great. Access to a psychologist, psychiatrist or medical clinic is simply not feasible for millions of people in rural, or impoverished, areas. I envision a world where peer workers provide psychiatric therapy, and low dose oral ketamine, to the most remote of villages. Ketamine is used as a 'buddy' drug in the battlefield; it has been injected by American soldiers, in Vietnam, Afghanistan and Iraq.

A soldier, severely wounded in the field will receive a ketamine injection, e.g., after an attack with an IED—improvised explosive device. Now at risk for PTSD and phantom limb pain, ketamine ought to be offered ketamine early on, *before* PTSD and neuropathy overwhelm the central nervous system. British and more recently, US Emergency Services are using ketamine, and in Australia it's the go-to medication for the Royal Flying Doctor Service.[35] From a humanitarian perspective, IM ketamine and a Toradol injection ought to be offered immediately, when someone with an intractable affliction and severe flare-up presents to an ER.[36]

* * *

In the US we've focused primarily on IV treatment, which requires closer supervision in outpatient clinics and hospitals, with blood pressure measurements and EKGs. It's effective, but ketamine IV treatments are cost prohibitive for many patients. For treatment resistant depression, and severe to intractable pain, any Primary Care Provider, psychiatrist or psychologist, can order oral or intranasal ketamine for a patient from a compounding pharmacy.

Ketamine has the potential to prevent acute pain from becoming chronic, thus avoiding permanent brain changes and *central sensitization*—a situation in which a patient's brain and spinal cord are permanently on high alert for distressing signals. Depression and other neuropsychiatric disorders change brain matter, too. Consider the geographical and socioeconomic situation in the United States and the barriers to care: how many people have quick access to a therapist, social worker or Pain Management clinic?

For a variety of reasons, we may have more in common with developing nations than we'd like to admit. So, why not provide patients oral ketamine, in the form of *troches*, while waiting for an anti-depressant to kick in, or to a patient with serious physical suffering, while they save money for an infusion or await prior authorization for an inpatient treatment? It's impossible for a patient to fill their oral ketamine prescription early. Most towns of a million souls may have at most three licensed compounding pharmacies; and they'd quickly alarm the prescriber.

One caveat, and a familiar complaint of chronic pain patients, is the associated fatigue and extreme exhaustion. Personally, this feeling of having a perpetual flu, is almost more debilitating than my neurological complaints. It's an awful, undertreated side effect and may be the result of fighting neuropathy or other chronic pain, on a daily basis. I address the topic of exhaustion briefly in the Practical Advice section, but surely will contemplate and write more about this topic the next book.

* * *

The Queen of Ketamine is a truthful, gritty account of struggling with physical agony and disability, and ultimately, becoming a comedian and writer. A couple of names have been changed to protect the privacy of those depicted, and in two cases, locations and identifying circumstances, as requested. Dialogue has been created from memory, medical notes, diaries, letters and three college size comedy notebooks.

This memoir/practical advice guide aims to provide hope and inspiration. Not hope in the sense that life as you once knew it will return, but that a pragmatic approach, and insight into your medical situation, may lead to a better quality of life. Should you suffer from adhesive arachnoiditis, cauda equina damage or central neuropathic pain, know that essentially, you have a type of spinal cord injury (SCI), spinal cord nerve root damage or rather, *spinal cord injury clinical syndrome.*[37]

You might need support the same way a patient with a complete SCI or CES needs rehabilitation, mobility aids, or household help. Likewise, for patients with CRPS or other diseases, you may benefit from Occupational and Physical Therapy. Unfortunately, 80 percent of patients with a complete, or an incomplete SCI, will develop neuropathic pain as well.

Although I have provided links and extensive footnotes to spruce up an argument, and have written everything as accurately as possible, this book should not be interpreted as research or medical advice. Always consult your medical team and provider. Disclaimer: my native language is Dutch, and I speak with a very pleasant, mild accent. Although my English is eloquent, it is inevitable that occasionally, Dutch-isms appear. All Italics in this book, including those within quotes, are my responsibility.

* * *

According to the National Institutes of Mental Health, neuropsychiatric disorders are the leading cause of disability; mental and behavioral disorders first, followed by neurological diseases—furthermore, back, neck pain and musculoskeletal disorders.[38] This human, and societal, cost will burden our medical network to a breaking point, in which alternatives to suffering must be sought out. Time is of the essence, especially with a rapidly aging population, since the number of patients with neuropathy may escalate in the future, as emphasized and explained in "Welcome to Hell."

With greater awareness and access to this life saving—and life changing treatment—we may give one and another a fighting chance. Imagine our individual journeys in this short life; voyages filled with hope, connection and creativity instead of never-ending despair. My basic belief, and main reason for writing this memoir, is that you deserve a better quality of life, no matter what your chronic medical or mental health problems are. Thus, I hope *The Queen of Ketamine* may serve as a fine companion to you.

Like many who became disabled, I sometimes still mourn for the loss of my career, and the person I was four, five years ago. This battle nearly did me in, and there is no conclusive happy ending. Since my skydiving accident,

I have fought valiantly for my health, and an identity other than that of a patient. Seems my failures outweigh my successes, yet life itself has been, and continues to be, worth living. I'm much more at peace than I was in 2015 and feel less lonely. And that's progress.

Albuquerque, December 2019

PART ONE

Peter Duke Photography, Santa Monica Pier

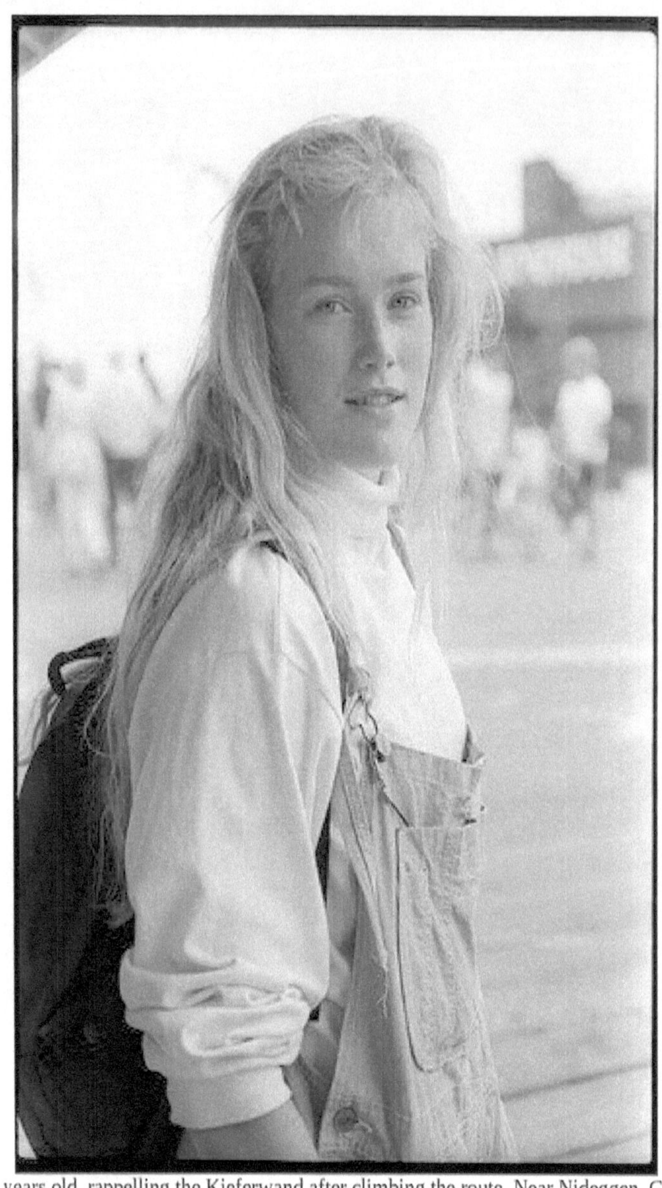

Seven years old, rappelling the Kieferwand after climbing the route. Near Nideggen, Germany

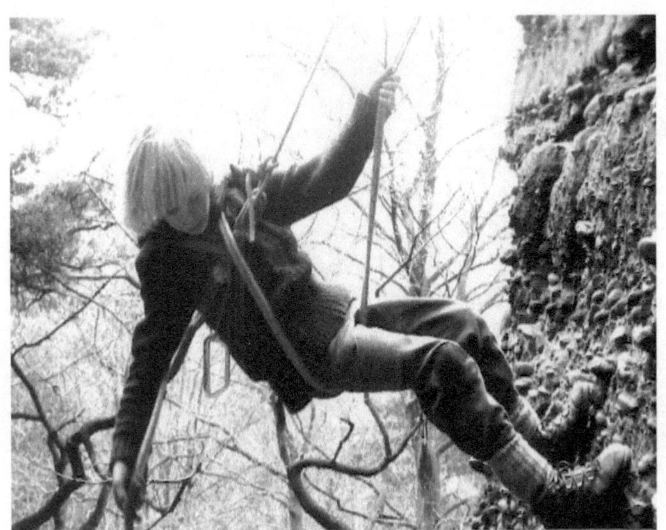

About a week before my accident.

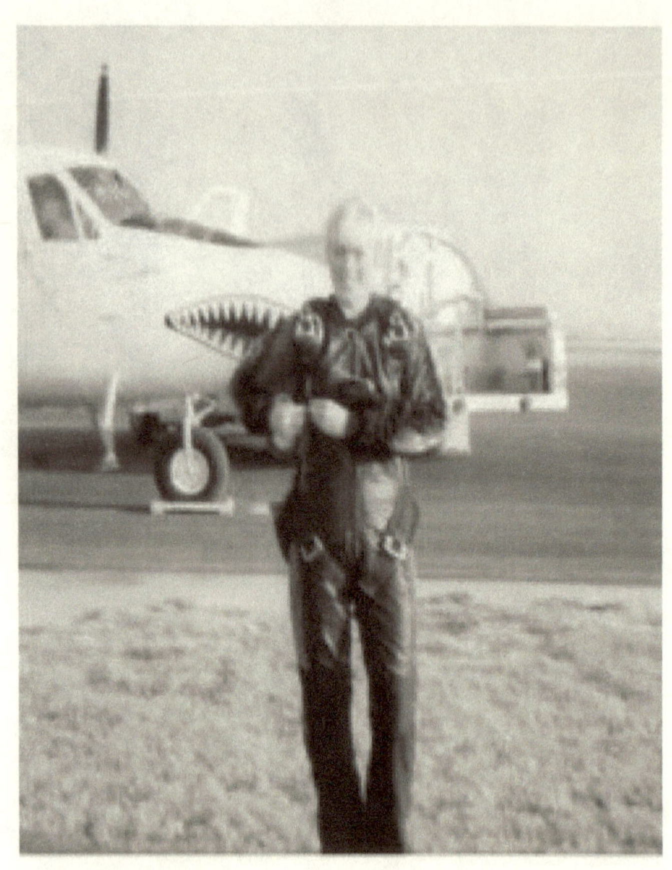

Perris Valley. The plane is a Twin Otter.

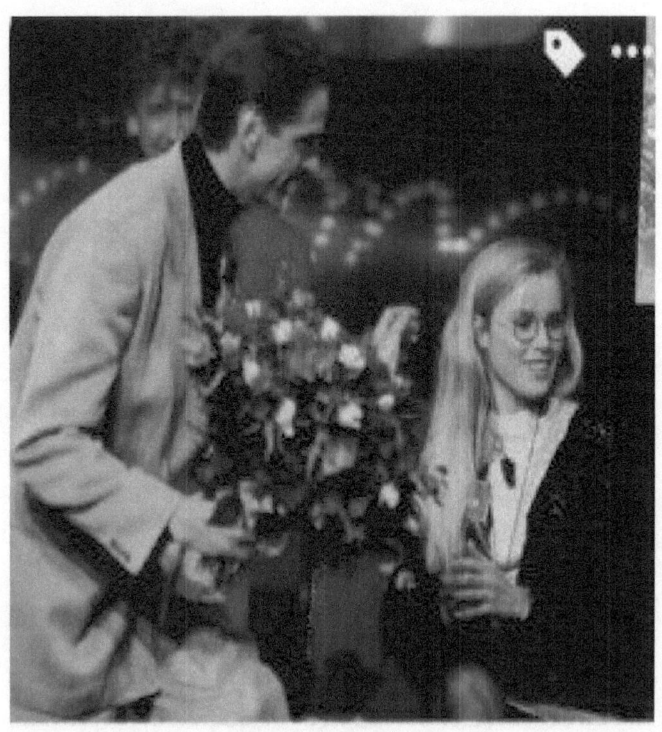

Jeremy Irons and I in a Dutch TV show.

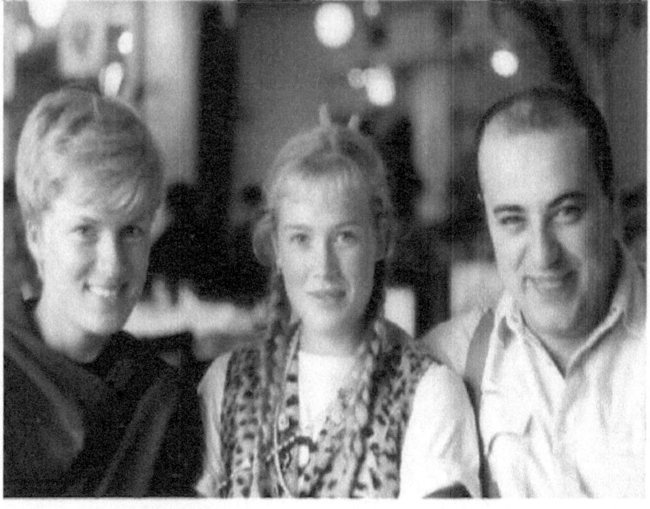

With Pascale Allione and Daniel Adjadj in a Parisian brasserie.
Naive but happy, this is what I looked like when Prince and I met.

1 READY, SET, GO!

"Gravity, thou art a heartless bitch." - Dr. Sheldon Cooper, The Big Bang Theory

October 10, 1992

I
t's a beautiful evening in the desert outside Los Angeles at Skydive Perris. The air smells sweet and expectant. Kerosene droplets and tiny particles of sand float around the runway, an invisible cloud in the innocuous, silken sky. The molecular mist, like a stealth army, creeps into my nostrils, and the delicate mucosa of my olfactory pathway relays the chemicals' presence throughout my neurons. The reptilian part of my brain screams alarm, but my inner adrenaline junkie loves it. The old DC-10 has finished refueling, and its outline appears cartoon-like against the dying rays, a beautiful, surreal sunset. The low-frequency vibrations of its engines pulsate through my bright orange earplugs.

I'm using my friend Charlie's rig. It's an older, square parachute—a compact package that covers my lovely, strong spine. My precious, beautiful brain, with its' underutilized neocortex, is protected only by the thin leather of a classic, aviator-style helmet, something Amelia Earhart would have worn in 1932. A black and purple polyester jumpsuit wreathes my muscular, boyish body. Underneath this outer cover, I'm wearing my favorite ratty, black T-shirt, the one with a white Jack Daniels bottle—ironic as I hardly ever drink—paired with stretchy cotton leggings. The grey leggings were a gift from a creepy old guy in Miami who once sent my friend Erica clothes from his sports label. Erica always got free gifts and free meals. Sigh.

I'm nauseated. I don't know if it's from fear, the smell of kerosene, or the half-eaten Seven Layer Taco Bell burrito I wolfed down on my way across the tarmac. Dave, the Jumpmaster, is waiting at the door to the plane, doing last-minute safety checks on two fellow skydivers who, like me, are geared up for their first nighttime jump. Dave's in his mid-to-late forties, and he looks ancient to my 24-year-old eyes. His thin, longish, blond hair waves in the propeller draft; I notice his belly stretches his jumpsuit in places where it shouldn't.

"Are you ready?" he asks.

"Yeah!" I answer, quickly throwing the rest of my burrito into the trash can. I hate wasting food.

Before I can board, he attaches a neon green glow stick over my altimeter —diagonally, so I can see my opening altitude. The altimeter itself is attached to a small, 45-degree-angled pillow, held by straps across my chest. All I must do is look down to read it when I'm flying through the sky.

Inside the plane, there's a group of about 20 additional skydivers, waiting for the three of us first-time night divers and our Jumpmaster to climb aboard. Like our trio, most of them will be doing individual dives, albeit at higher altitude. There's also a D-level team that will be doing more advanced group formations. Because us newbies will jump from a lower altitude, we're last in and first out.

Dave completes our safety checks while adjusting straps and issuing final instructions. We're to exit the plane at 7,500 feet and open our parachutes at 2,500. Panic stirs deep in my gut. I normally open at a much more conservative 3,500 feet. In my mind, I repeat some rough calculations.

Let's see; gravity and the speed of acceleration will have me plunging toward the ground at 32 feet per second, squared. If I were to exit the plane at 7,500 feet and jump without a parachute, it would take about 46 or 47 seconds to hit the ground. The first 1,000 feet will take 10, 11 seconds, then acceleration will increase until every 1000 feet takes only five seconds. By then, I'll be traveling at terminal velocity, 120 miles per hour. Around 31 seconds after exiting the plane I will pull my ripcord, at 2,500 feet.

By my calculations, the timed difference between opening at 3,500 and 2,500 feet is only five seconds, but if something goes wrong, five extra seconds to pull the reserve and land safely seems huge. At Jumpmaster Dave's 2,500 feet, we have little time to adjust for error, and a lot can go right—or wrong—in those few moments. My throat constricts, and a feeling of doom settles in my chest.

"You okay?" Dave asks, grabbing my harness for final inspection. My inner voice screams in terror, but not a single sound crosses my lips. Chronic low self-esteem, one of my default settings, renders me mute. I already feel like a fraud in general, and I decide not to announce my unease. Swallowing my fear is a small price to pay for earning my C-level certification, and this nighttime jump is the final piece. Deciding I'll do what the man says, I climb on board with my fellow skydivers.

* * *

Earlier that day, Bad Spot Bill had plowed some 16-foot-wide target circles to soften the desert hardpan, creating little dirt "cushions" for our touchdowns. He's out at the landing zone now with John Restivo, his mechanic friend, who'll be overseeing our descent. Guided by their truck lights, we can aim ourselves at the target circles we'd otherwise not find in the darkness. This comforts me somewhat.

I always land the mark. With 58 daytime jumps under my belt, the six most recent have been with Skydive Perris; so far, Bad Spot Bill has never had to track *me* down in the desert because of an off-target landing. I may have had a mediocre modeling career and been fired recently from my job as a TV presenter, but if I keep moving toward my goal of becoming a fulltime stuntwoman, I feel invincible.

I know there's a stiffness about me; it comes from a fear that courses through my limbs, my blood, my youth. It kept me from dancing until I was 18. It took me seven years to feel somewhat comfortable in front of the camera. At a shoot in Milan, famed Benetton photographer Olivero Toscani had once accused me of moving "like a garbage can" and he fired me from his photography studio. Although he was an asshole, he was probably right. I did have all the grace of moving like a garbage can, except when I was flying through space.

All those years of modeling had made me feel as though I were merely a head, adorned with a too-symmetrical face framed by long, strawberry blonde hair; a head attached to a body, a body that moved through space aimlessly. Nothing I had experienced while modeling let me connect my beautiful athleticism to my inquisitive mind or to my courageous soul. Photographers and their cameras reduced me to a mechanism for selling merchandise, a sexual object. Smile. Turn. Chin down. Chin up. Make sexy eyes. Despite their insistence, I never could flirt with the camera or, as I had seen others do, with my photographers.

My aversion to the camera didn't improve after a brief stint as a television broadcaster, earlier this year. I quickly learned that what I hate even more than modeling is speaking through a microphone or being filmed as myself. Or some version of myself. I hate my voice, so soft and insecure sounding.

The TV opportunity as a sports reporter came about because I'd been searching for a way out of my modeling career, which had been miserable, at best. That "best" was when I connected with a nice team—which wasn't often enough—or when I modeled sports clothes, especially mountaineering, the demanding sport I had done since childhood. I loved that part. What I do not actively despise about my body are my legs. Now, my feet are nothing to look at, no photographer ever took pictures of my ugly toes in a pretty sandal. But my legs ought to be immortalized in a marble statue, they're a piece of art, so strong.

* * *

Once, I came out of a Belgian forest after a pee, when I was camping with my older friends. During the day, we scaled thousand-feet cliffs, at night we got high and entertained each other with rock climbing and hitchhiking adventures. Wading through the moist, tall grasses in the dark, heading back to my tent I'd glanced down, the moon lighting up my pale, shorts-cladded legs. I was suddenly in awe, of how much I loved my legs.

And now, my newfound career as a stuntwoman and these powerful, muscular legs will give me the best of both worlds. I can indulge in my travel addiction, and I can keep flooding my daredevil brain with adrenaline.

Oh, and let's not forget the food!

I'm not much of a cook and relied on the photography studios' lunches and buffets. On trips, the generous per diems guaranteed the easy eating provided by restaurant chefs or room service. As a stuntwoman working for Dutch movies and television, I'd already experienced great catering. However, being a stuntwoman in the Netherlands wasn't going to lead to a full-time career.

So, without my weekly TV job, I left for America and relocated to Los Angeles, where they make plenty of movies. Why wouldn't I make it in Hollywood, doing stunts for a living? I knew I was no Jeannie Epper, but figured I'd give it a shot. Gerard Depardieu, after meeting me in Costa Rica, had said to his stuntman buddy Nick Gillard (who introduced us): "She has the eyes of a bullfighter!" His compliment was way better than getting yelled at by photographer Olivero Toscani— and his ilk—for moving like a stiff.

I'm principled and try to avoid rich people as much as I can. In my heart of hearts, I feared they'd only ever see my outer appearance. They'd never understand my stubbornness or mountaineering ways. That's why I'm not going to the party tonight, that my friend Clara had invited me to. Her parents, famous musician Jean Luc Ponty and his wife, own a beautiful home near the ocean in Santa Monica. I felt that the ways of Hollywood and its social nuances are lost on me and refused to mingle with wealth or fame. I didn't even bother going to the wrap party Nick had invited me to.

Remembering my graceless demise at the Dutch television station a few months earlier, I think: *Wow, I don't burn bridges; I napalm the shit out of them. I definitely do not belong to the confident, successful and beautiful crowd.* I'd discovered that TV producer John H. accepted cash money under the table by a nightclub owner, to shoot there for publicity. I wrote an indignant letter about the lack of journalistic integrity and, of course, was promptly fired.

* * *

Tonight, this skydive, will change everything. This night jump will give me my C license, the second highest rating, and I may be able to specialize in skydiving stunts. I will be admired for my daring ways, not for my outward, photogenic appearance. I can leave behind the itchy catalog sweaters, posing for the camera, and being trussed up by high heels and short skirts. Never mind that, even as a stuntwoman, I've been cast as the pretty, skimpily clad girl doing stunt fights in bars. Never mind that 2,500-foot conundrum waiting for me ahead.

Like a sailor lost at sea, clinging to a piece of wood from a shipwreck, I cling to the promise of the C license; it is my ticket to liberation from the superficial, petty denizens of Tinseltown and the Modeling Mafia. Instead of telling Jumpmaster Dave that I'd rather not pull at 2,500 feet, I stare out the dirty, oval window. Revealed below, a lonely stretch of desert where once there flowed an inland sea. Now, like most of the Southwest, the granite bedrock is covered with soil.

The other skydivers are busy prepping, and the D-Level team is gesturing to one another as they rehearse the complicated moves they'll be doing in sync. I wish I were on their skydiving team. A few of them grace with me with nods and smiles and I suddenly miss my teammates from Midden-Zeeland Skydiving Club.

Before I moved to the States, after years of a wandering, rather solitary existence, I had finally discovered community among their ranks. Jan, my Dutch skydiving instructor, and his daughter, Monique, an accomplished skydiver herself, had been such wonderful support for me in my newfound passion these last few months. It hits me: my time with the Midden Zeeland team was the best summer of my life.

I hug my knees; my eyes tear up behind my goggles.

Only six months ago, 16 skydivers, two of whom belonged to the Dutch 'Tomscat' team, had died in a horrendous plane crash at this Perris airfield. Monique's fiancée, Remi, was among them. Her poor father, Jan, the sweet, stocky contractor who has taught me so much, had lost his only son a few years earlier during a skydiving course. It had been his son's eighth skydive. When I was training with them, I hadn't realized that underneath Jan and Monique's warm and easy demeanor there was so much sorrow.

* * *

Oh God, the heartache! As one of the two deadliest sports—the other hang gliding—it's the dirty, hidden secret. Falling from the sky, bodies littering the planet; landing in trees, electricity lines, on rock, gravel, and grass. Predominantly, those broken bodies belonged to young people, exchanging an adrenaline-filled lifestyle for a coffin—or a wheelchair.

I don't have time to think about that right now. Besides, death and disease won't happen to me. Instead, I'll become a full-time, professional stuntwoman and work with stunt coordinators who matter, like Dickey Beer —who'd hired me already. I'd met and worked alongside Vic Armstrong, who coordinated Spielberg movies, and his cute and cocky friend, Nick Gillard. My goodness, even working as a stand-in would give me access to catering, good food and an unlimited supply of Diet Coke!

I tremble with the excitement, the ripples of time moving around me like water caressing a stone in a wild and unruly river. As if I can touch, feel and smell the possibilities of this endless Universe. Taking a cue from the D team divers, I mentally rehearse my upcoming maneuvers, step-by-step, from up here in the Heavens all the way down to Planet Earth. First, I'll do a simple tumble in the sky, as I've successfully done a dozen times before. Afterward, I will check my altimeter and pull my chute at 2,500 instead of 3,500 feet, as agreed.

The steep ascent is over, and the DC10's engine sound different, now that we've reached 7500 feet she is coasting for a bit. The airplane door opens and cold air, vaguely salty, swooshes around the cabin. Ah, adrenaline! It's time. Nothing bad will ever happen to me. Jumpmaster Dave is next to the opening, signaling me to come over. I stand at the precipice, and he and I count together:

"Ready!"

"Set."

"Go!"

And I go, diving into darkness. Long, strawberry blonde braids swirl and whip around my face, while my body floats above the desert, finding its equilibrium with an arched back. In the distance, Lake Elsinore reflects a luminous, beautiful moon, a beacon of hope for humanity. The adrenaline rush is magnificent, and I've never felt more at home than I do at this moment. I belong to the sky. Although I'll be back on earth in less than a minute, I'm reveling in this brief, peak experience.

I check the altimeter, and I'm at 3,500 feet; I bite back the temptation to do what instinct and training taught me. My silence, now a promise, shores up my resolve to wait another 5 seconds to pull. I take one breath and let it out. I draw a breath in and pull the ripcord.

Under most circumstances, it takes about three seconds for the chute to fully deploy and feel the harsh jolt of a slowing descent. We're taught to count it out.

One, one thousand (this is going well);

Two, one thousand (where's the string above me);

Three, one thousand (where's the jolt);

Four, one thousand (uh-oh, starting to twirl around, like a cheap pinata parachute toy).

Oh, shit. I shouldn't be spinning around and around like I'm on one of those carnival rides with swings suspended on chains. There must be a line crossing the chute canopy; full deployment isn't going to happen.

This isn't a carnival ride. This is a parachute malfunction of the worst kind. I'm in a "spinning mall," or, in skydiving parlance, the "spin of death." I check my altimeter, and it reads 1,500.

Another second, gone. I have only six, maybe seven seconds left to live.

There's only one thing to do now: decide to drop the main or leave it on and pull the reserve.

Jan hammered it into my muscle memory: above 1,000 feet, ditch the main, then pull the reserve to avoid entanglement. Below 1,000 feet, pull the reserve and hope for the best.

Disoriented, dizzy, and panicky, I look down again at the altimeter, but I can't see the 1,000-foot mark because there's this neon green glowstick covering the dial. Am I at 1,100? 1,000? Or 900? I don't know.

Death is imminent.

My life is not complete.

I'm not ready to die.

One more second, gone. The altimeter reading doesn't matter. In one panicked, fluid motion—and what my heroes Bad Spot Bill and John Restivo will later describe as the fastest maneuver they've ever seen—I drop the defunct main and simultaneously pull the ripcord for my reserve.

I have 400 feet—one last second—left.

There is only darkness.

***

I'm lying in the Perris Valley desert. The blackness, registering through my flickering eyelids, is punctuated by shiny bits of light. The stars. Then the moon. A few minutes ago, I interpreted its presence as a beacon of hope for humanity. Now that beacon is only a small, white circle, cut sharply from the black velvet cloth that envelops me. Seems a bleak universe, with mostly black matter, surrounds my existence.

I am a sack of bones, a leaking vessel. My arteries and veins no longer contain the necessary five liters of life-sustaining, precious blood. My once beautiful skeleton and essential bones are reduced to dozens and dozens of fragments, some as small as the period at the end of this sentence.

I hear voices, shouting at me, "Keep breathing!"

Bad Spot Bill and John Restivo try to carefully remove my aviator helmet. Suddenly, the identity I created in the preceding two and a half decades, the one I was trying to escape, is something I desperately want. I try even harder to reclaim what is forever lost. *I really should have gone to Clara's party…it is all my fault.* My mind, the one thing I've counted on over the years, is a dandelion, its tufts violently dispersed by the breath of a rambunctious child.

Again, I hear voices, yelling, "Keep breathing!"

I breathe. To draw a single breath, I grunt frantically, like when I used to harpoon ice axes into frozen waterfalls, pulling myself up, only to harpoon again. Ice climbing is one of the most challenging sports; drawing a simple breath now is even harder.

I'm too aware that my legs, once my two-pronged source of pride and joy as well as my symbol of personal freedom, are gone. My skull holds my precious brain. How much of it is left intact in there? My tailbone and lower back, upon which I landed, feels smashed into a million pieces. My heart is beating too rapidly and soon merges with the deep *whoop, whoop* of a rescue helicopter. I know the sound too well, from past mountaineering expeditions, and it is always the sound of doom.

Oh, come on, guys, I think. *Cancel the trauma chopper, because I've lived in this "new" body for a full 10 minutes now, and I'm over it. This is not going to end well.*

My sense of self scattered, my thoughts flushed away like water after a torrential rainstorm, a temporary river careening through a desert arroyo. *Water always searches for the lowest point, going back to where life began.* I take short, staccato breaths as my fractured ribs pierce my lungs, which are filling up fast. Feels like I'm drowning and choking on my own blood.

I gasp for air like a prehistoric fish, washed ashore from the ancient sea that once covered this desert floor. Geological forces millennia ago altered this landscape, rendering it permanently changed, as I now am. I am condemned to live in the Land of the Sick and Crippled, and there is no return ticket. My passport to freedom is revoked. And I taste the sickening iron, the metal in my mouth, and every breath and meek cough torments me, ails me so that I wish for death, after all.

* * *

My mind mixes this horrifying truth with the unfolding, surreal tableau. Like a big Hollywood production, everyone around me is playing their role to perfection. The bystanders, the medics, the courageous chopper pilot, my two heroes Bad Spot Bill and John Restivo, who moved their truck so I wouldn't land on it.

A million to one odds though: when I bounced three feet into the air the first time after hitting the ground, I happened to land inside that 16-foot-diameter circle of softer, recently plowed earth instead of the concrete like, hard desert. That plowed circle saved my life. I never miss my mark, and this landing was no exception.

As my demolished body is loaded onto the stretcher, the moon I'd admired when I was flying looks down on the scene, cold and uncaring. My legs are engulfed by wave after wave of worsening agony as trauma pants are inflated. There's an oxygen mask over my face. With my tailbone and vertebral fractures, lying immobilized on a flat hardboard hurts so much more. It feels as if my body had been ripped in half.

They load me into the chopper and then, back up into the night sky I go. Inside the noisy, vibrating trauma helicopter, the paramedics treat me as just another body to keep alive. My chest, with its cracked ribs and blood-filled lungs, burns with something other than ache. Shame, guilt, and fears of future gossip: *Of course, it was her own fault! She always took too many risks!*

The African American paramedic yells, "72 over 50," while she checks on both IVs, one for each arm. A defibrillator stands nearby. She quickly confirms the trauma pants are fully inflated. They push blood toward my heart to keep me alive. I gasp through the mask and feel the oxygen push painfully into my half-inflated lungs. The humming from the trauma chopper goes straight through my body, and I sense every oscillating turn of the blades. This new hell hurts me in more ways than I ever imagined. I shouldn't have survived.

Instead of gently flowing out into nothingness and death, after yet another nauseating wave of pain, I give it one more shot and try to survive the next few breaths. *Fucking hell, I'm in my beloved America, my chosen homeland, and if I survive, it's because of the American soldiers on the battlefield. Most trauma protocol originates from the Korean and Vietnam Wars…aren't they supposed to shoot me up with morphine about now?* I am drowning in an ocean of suffering. I'm in shock, but that isn't numbing the ache enough. I struggle to draw yet another breath and have a flashback of my past life.

Once, on a fashion shoot to the Seychelles, an American model pushed me into the pool, while the entire team cheered her on. I was wearing a sad, cheap cotton evening dress, which clung to my 17-year-old, flat-chested skinny body. I felt so humiliated, and defenseless, and the next day, my tormenter stole my only lipstick, and smoked cigarettes in the non-smoking room we shared. The cheek!

The American beauty thought she was so hot, she should "play the lead for the *Lucky* film adaptation," one of those fun, trashy mid-eighties books Jackie Collins deftly wrote. On that same trip, a kind hotel maid, Malika, had invited me into the jungle. We spoke and laughed in French while she taught me to pick verbena leaves for tea. I'd learned repeatedly that my friendly demeanor mostly endeared me to hotel maids and janitors. Although I did have a few photographer and modeling friends, I never seemed part of their world.

And I liked it that way.

Now, seething with self-hatred, and filled with deep regret, I didn't know how to face a future without my legs. I need them to escape society, and mean people. Perhaps, if life wants me to play this silly game of life and death, I know what my role entails. I'll pretend again—this time to be a grateful survivor, a model patient.

Soft, muddled sounds come out of my blood-smeared mouth, "I'm. . . so sorry," I say through the oxygen mask, trying to make eye contact with the medic.

"What?!" she answers, while looking at the EKG, "Keep quiet, we're almost there!"

"I'm so sorry I can't enjoy this ride. Because I really love helicopters," I say in a harsh, loud whisper. The paramedics and trauma chopper pilot seem quite determined to deliver me to Riverside General alive, but I wonder: *What if, by rescuing me, they are condemning me to a fate much, much worse than death?*

2 NOT BORN ON AMERICAN SOIL/HINTERLANDS

I never let schooling interfere with my education. - Mark Twain, author & humorist

Holland. Such a small, lovely, green country; a marvel of social engineering, equal amounts of democracy and monarchy. I couldn't wait to leave those flat lands, although I have a terrible weakness for sparkling mountain streams, glaciers, rivers and large bodies of water. What sane person wouldn't? On the other hand, there's something compelling about the empty, harsh beauty of the American Southwest desert. Growing up, it seemed as though a piece of my soul was missing, or maybe I did not feel deserving of the lush Dutch landscape. Not that I believe in a soul, being raised atheist. Despite not being able to fully leave my past behind me—I love Ikea and European tidiness—there was something special about America.

Pretty sure I'm gonna die. This is my earliest memory, another one was kicking the backyard barbecue when I was mad, lost that fight. During a hiking holiday in the French Alps, I had fallen ill with a high fever, and was medevaced into the valley, from high above the tree line. The ramblings of the old Jeep truck shook me to my bones as we raced down steep mountain curves, the ravine to the left yearning for us to fall into. My mother and I were in the back, in the open air, with yellow and green ponchos against the rain. Our backpacks were wet and with every turn on that steep, primitive trail, I thought we'd tumble in the deep nothingness below.

I was four, and finally old enough to go mountaineering with my parents. I was glad, because they had left me alone for two to three weeks every year since I was born. Well, with friends or family, but I sure was happy to be a big girl and join their adventures. My parents each had waxed cotton backpacks; belongings such as a first aid kit, cookware, food and gas stove meticulously stowed inside. Maps went in the zippered compartment on top, water bottles and sunscreen in the side pockets.

We wore knickerbockers, pants just below the knee, one pair of long, thin stockings underneath shorter, grey wool socks inside leather, handstitched Dachsteins, an Austrian mountaineering boot. As I got older, I feared that younger, cooler looking climbers would laugh at our family, clad in quintessential 1930's outfit. Carabiners, ropes and other items were stowed on top for easy access, as we often traversed fields of snow, ice, and rock walls. My parents wielded a long, wooden pickaxe with a metal tool on top, which they held in whatever hand was closest to a steeply iced, rock or snowclad mountain side.

Ideally, in case of a fall, they were to throw themselves flat against the frozen snow, belly first, legs apart to slow down, then jam the pickaxe into the hardened snow. I suspect they were just for show; since we were all attached to one another by rope, we would most likely perish and slide down into a death. It's not that I didn't trust my parents, who you know, gave me food—although never enough—and shelter after a ten-hour hike. It's that nature will always win, except that time we outran a huge snow avalanche coming at us in the Julian Alps.

I felt at home in the most majestic of landscapes, yet knew myself to be miniscule, maybe because of those mountains. Given our perilous, yet exciting mountaineering expeditions, I was also bored as fuck back home, in the lowlands. I had three coping strategies: stuffing my face with candy, reading and 'kattekwaad uithalen' aka getting into trouble. Sometimes, even doing all three at once, would not fill that gaping abyss in my heart. My favorite havoc causing method was running away. As a young toddler, they had me in a wooden corral, but I quickly figured out that stacking all the toys gave me enough leverage to escape. Hey, I was top dog in my wooden kiddie coral.

By age seven, I'd escape to my favorite junkyard and climb on top of cars stacked eight high, eating melted chocolates and browsing rained on porn magazines, or reading a small Penguin book. It was heaven, being alone in the hinterlands. This was my world, my domain, and no one could tell me what to do. Of course, I was wracked by guilt when I finally came home after sundown. My stomach led me straight to the dining table, but as punishment, I was sent up to my small room. After an hour of sulking in the dark, my father came up, bringing toast with apple syrup, which I despised. *I am seven years old, and he still doesn't know I loathe the thick, gooey apple syrup that tastes like iron? This is no olive branch, this is an insult!* I threw the toast towards his back in the doorway, the interaction leaving both of us in a well rage.

* * *

Growing up, death was always violent and unexpected, it was nothing like seeing a beloved grandparent resting peacefully in a coffin. Mountaineering took us to Italy, to climb the magnificent Brenta Dolomites in Italy. It was supposed to be my last innocent summer, before boys started pinching my budding breasts, and we would lose the first of three Scouting friends, Anita, to leukemia. As usual, I had a lot on my twelve-year-old mind when we were hiking, least of all my confusion, after seeing Treat Williams in *Hair*. That man was fit. And I'd really liked Marco at Elementary School.

"Que dio mio!" the warden of 'Refugio' Pedrotti exclaimed sadly, upon hearing the hysterical yelling. (Strangely, I would yell the same words 'Oh my God!' three times, when I was plummeting to my death.) 'Refugio' is the Italian word for mountain hut. These huts range from primitive four wall shelter carved into granite to a two-story hostel with kitchen, but all featured outhouses and none had plumbing.

At 2491 meters, Refugio Pedrotti was spectacularly set, far above the tree line, surrounded by serrated mountains and gigantic, almost ninety-degree rock walls with a gigantic field of smaller pebbles, remnants from ancient glaciers. From a geophysical perspective, the Brenta Dolomites are a 'younger' mountain range at only a few hundred million years and thus, appeared sharper and more hostile than the Colorado plateau. The tectonic plates that forced rocks towards the heavens created razor sharp, fear inspiring peaks, and therefore, some of the best technical climbing routes, which attracted young, agile climbers.

Screams pierced the clear and odorless morning air—just the way I liked air to smell, without the screams of course. Mountain mornings are always cold, breathing hurts a little, but the outside air is fresh, whereas inside the hut is like all others; an olfactory assault of wet, dank socks, sweat, farts and coffee. And wood fire. There are no paths to this hut except metal ladders, an iron network—Via Ferrata—and narrow trails, supplies are flown in by helicopter. This is, for all practical purposes, the end of the world. There are no other children except for my brother and sister, which I like too.

Back home, I quickly realized most of my cohorts—the other kids in nursery and kindergarten seemed fucking useless—with their incessant whining and lack of focus. Worst of all, they resorted to some serious Lord of the Flies shit; to either alienate me from the few friends I had, or to get me to kowtow to their warlord bitch. (Although I was also extremely sensitive, and my parents hadn't prepared me well for life along other humans.) I'd observed some adults that seemed a little more sensible so had high hopes for the future. On the other hand, here I was, stuck with my hapless parents. By the time I was nine, I knew I could do a much better job raising myself. *Amateur hour is over, folks!* I longed for my own identity, away from my family; yet, I was overcome with shame, guilt, and homesickness whenever I wanted to be by myself.

Here in the mountains though, there is a kind of solitude and zero bullying, although there's a higher probability of death and I'm with my family 24/7. In life, there's always a tradeoff, you can't have it all. The Via Ferrata is conquered with a climbing harness, and a short rope extending from that harness with two karabiners on each of the ends. One gets clicked onto the ladder spurt, or a metal cable on the wall, and slowly, ensuring that at all time, at least one carabiner is clipped in, I secure myself going up. Did I already mention that beneath us is a 500 meters—1640 feet—abyss to die in? My younger siblings have an additional safety rope attached to my parents' harness, but I am almost thirteen. We clip in and out, on metal ladders and horizontal ledges, all day long.

* * *

I'd started *visiting the bat cave* that Spring and was petrified of being found out. Despite all the progressive magazines for young teenagers with cover articles such as "You go, girl, self-pleasuring is normal!" I was so embarrassed. Surely, I was the only person in the world having lewd thoughts —although they were mediocre compared to the stash my friend and I would later find. She was *so* lucky to have two older brothers. At the same time, since it seemed purely physical sensation, I had no desire to share this icky, bodily stuff with another human. Enough about *ménage à moi*, let's get back to death.

The warden, now mad with frustration, stamped his feet as the screams became more desperate, amplified from the nearly vertical, 2000-foot rock wall across the rocky field. His felt hat was crooked, his cheeks bright red, and he was yelling at his cook and helper to radio for the rescue team. The screaming must have come from the technical climbers, who explored new routes and traced the hardest climbs, above the Via Ferrata. A small figure was lying down, silent. That made sense, it's only the living that yell their lungs out—unless you have blood in them and just landed at 70 mph, then it's a soft whisper.

The helicopter crew rescued the young French climber, then went back to pick up his girlfriend's corpse, which was now swinging underneath the helicopter like a pendulum. The warden had to identify the body, as the sole survivor was in shock. "It's my 21st body, I can't do this no more!" he allegedly said, translated by an Austrian mountaineer. The climber's grey, terror-stricken face made him seem twice as old. It was my fault we'd witness this tragedy: we had already tried leaving Refugio Pedrotti a few hours ago.

My father was on a tight schedule while guiding his wife and children through the mountains, along routes painstakingly determined and researched during the long Dutch winter months. The day before had been especially strenuous, that morning I'd felt physically, and psychologically, exhausted. One could be physically sick but not mentally, so a tummy ache was an acceptable reason to return to the Refugio Pedrotti. We'd only hiked for 30 minutes, after the Herculean task of getting the five of us ready, fed, and packed up for the day ahead.

I ended up taking pictures of the rescue helicopter, and the body dangling underneath, then put some yellow flowers at the shed where the climber's body rested. My father collected 30 feet of photo albums, but my pictures did not appear anywhere, as if my memories of that day were extinguished. I wasn't even upset as there was no use arguing.

* * *

One of my very few one-liner jokes is that "I was raised without a father… but there was a misogynist who showed up for dinner every day at six." My dad was the Master of Mixed Signals, either angry, hostile and irritated by kids and women—who were of course, also terrible drivers—or he was overly sentimental and wanted his loyal battalion, us, to understand him. From my first breath, I've had the daunting sensation of being in the wrong place at the wrong time, or wrong decade, except when I was hiking, alone in the mountains. Or climbing on top of my kingdom, the junkyard.

Beyond our endless shouting matches which I lost because inevitably, I'd burst into tears—while my father regained power—there was the occasional smack across my face. Even at age fourteen in a Chinese restaurant, for all I knew I was *too loud* or had *misbehaved*. I never understood why, nor where my father's frustration with me came from. Behind his glacier-like blue eyes, there simmered a fiery volcano of rage that was quick to erupt. And it seemed he'd blamed me for his foul mood since I was a little kid.

Age fourteen, I ran away a few months later, spending the night with a buddy. When dad found me and dragged me home, he cried in the living room, his head bend in his hands. "You are the child that makes me the angriest and the one that makes me happiest. Why are you doing this to me?" he said, sobbing in his favorite, brown corduroy cladded armchair. No one asked why I had run away in the first place. In my early thirties I finally mustered up the courage to ask him why he'd smacked me in public as a teen. "Why?" he replied, "Who knows why. Some children just ask for it." My dad's reply had a kind of funny irony to it. But damn, he didn't even remember slapping me!

* * *

Despite all that, I loved our family and our idiosyncrasies; watching "Soap", "Fawlty Towers" and "The A-Team" in the spare TV time we were allocated, half an hour a day, and only two channels to choose from. Comedy and our wild and dangerous adventures created cohesion. How dangerous? We all wore dog tags. At first, I thought it was so we could send postcards to our two cats—the metal tags had our physical address. Hey, I was six. My dad then explained it was to reunite the family in case we were split, but since we were usually attached together by climbing gear and ropes, that made no sense either. Then I saw a Vietnam documentary with teenagers wearing dog tags just like mine, only a second later, to show bodies in a bag.

It finally dawned on me that we wore dog tags, so they'd know where to ship *our* bodies. Sometimes we'd drive through the night on our return trip home, from the mountains back to the flat Dutch landscape. Whether we arrived at midnight or 2:00 a.m., my father, perhaps relaxed and relieved that we were all alive, allowed us to unload, while he ran to the kitchen. He'd cook delicious, Dutch pancakes while we argued over who would get to read the new issue of Donald Duck first. We still had green, sour apples from our tiny orchard, and bacon, to mix with the batter.

The butter turned brown and dark, tufts of smoke rising, the air sticky and delicious, before the batter was poured into a cast iron pan the size of a large dinner plate. Topped off with real syrup, we knew what heaven tasted and smelled like, while my mom regaled us with her tales of running away all the way in the North, falling into a harbor or finding abandoned factories and her own hinterlands. But never joked about the months she was locked in a closet as a toddler, by an aunt and uncle.

My dad, a strait-laced, skeptical engineer also had a wicked sense of humor, though he leaned toward sarcasm. Dad would usually introduce himself to my friends as "Hi, I'm Kaatje's dad. Most likely." While perhaps two percent of children are not born from their mother's partner or spouse— the 10 percent figure of "bastard" children is an urban myth—there was no denying I was my father's daughter. I had his brains, his hands and fingers, and like him, I have never been a team player. I inherited my mom's strong, distinctive accent from the North, strangers would ask me if I was from Den Helder.

It is hard to fathom, but despite being born asphyxiated, with my mother's umbilical cord around my neck, surviving stone or snow avalanches with the family, outsmarting suburban pedophiles and exhibitionists—we call them "pencil venters" in Dutch, rock climbing without climbing gear or parental permission at age eight, diving into a ravine for a wild strawberry— my dad grabbing me just in time, breaking and entering, and setting car tires on fire, I made it through the first ten years of my life. Surviving my childhood was either an epic triumph of the human spirit, or luck. Yeah, definitely, luck.

* * *

In the summer of 1980, after a full day of high-altitude hiking in the Spanish Pyrenees, my family and I were stranded, among the bare rocks, glaciers, and snowfields atop the mountain range. Snowfields were always beautiful, exciting, and a tad terrifying because I didn't know if I would fall into a crevasse, the space where frozen snow and rock meets. Night was falling fast, and we needed shelter. A few hundred meters below, we came across a pair of shepherds, an old man and his nephew, living together in a forlorn, depressing mountain cabin. There was a tiny, decrepit attic where they said we could all sleep together.

While our little brother was playing outside, my sister Nicolien and I climbed the ladder to the small space, where we shook a pile of dust-caked blankets and cleared space for the seven of us. We choked and coughed, then laughed. The old man peaked in from the hole in the wooden floor, and suddenly yelled at us, in an unknown Spanish dialect. He was not happy about the two of us messing with his blankets.

The uncle was so upset, he threatened to kick us out, in the coldness of the dark night with nowhere to go. His nephew was in his early twenties but already missed several teeth, aged by a hard existence without running water and electricity. After some negotiation, the nephew insisted that my parents, sister, brother and I could spend the night but only if I kissed the grandpa. The grinning geezer stood next to his young charge, while staring at me with his good eye, the other moving around in the left socket, uncontrollably.

My parents negotiated peace and protected me by sleeping in between the senior citizen and I. Almost thirteen years old, I was naïve and innocent, and had never been kissed. According to my Dad, it was one of the more horrifying nights of his life. I assume that remained true until the night of the skydiving accident, when I was taken by trauma chopper to Riverside General with a fifty percent chance of making it.

Come to think of it, where were my parents when my little self was preyed upon by a nasty neighbor three doors down? He'd gesture for me to sit on his lap and whispered in my ear "you can only go home if you give me a kiss," in full view of his cowardly wife. It felt as if danger lurked everywhere. I did not enjoy being geriatric candy, although it would make for great jokes onstage. Unfortunately, despite being an overly rambunctious child, I was also raised to be polite. It might be best if little girls were taught kickboxing; turn them into adorable ninjas, and I bet global sexism and forced marriages would be eradicated, fast.

* * *

Much older and wiser, I've realized that despite my bad experiences, I was lucky not to be born during the Middle Ages. I would have been a very pretty peasant's daughter, and there's no doubt someone would have sold, abducted, or sent me away to satisfy a Duke, or perhaps, royalty. But I was a 20th century girl, and instead, my looks took me to the international modeling world, which one could argue isn't much better. And I *still* ended up acquainted with princes, first by meeting and befriending Prince, the musician, and then, Prince Albert of Monaco. What the heck was that about?

Overall, even if some adults were dangerous, as a child, their company meant a lot less bullying. Although that changed when I grew up and realized that too many of us treat life—and each other—like middle or high school kids. An educational psychologist had tested me at age eleven, and quickly determined "She suffers from crippling social and academic insecurities that have a detrimental effect on her ability to succeed. With professional help, she can learn to overcome this."

The referral was presumably instigated by Martin, my kindhearted elementary school teacher at the Rainbow School—I was bullied so badly at my first elementary school, they'd recommended switching schools when I was eight. Despite the report, my parents seemed to loathe psychiatrists and psychologists, and believed everything could be solved by going for a strenuous hike. Sadly, the bullying didn't stop, there were many other tormenters in my village.

While my mom was winning another tennis game barely ten meters away, in the bushes, I was outnumbered three to one. Against the loud, powerful sound of my mom's serve and tennis racket, my tormenters, from the rich area in town, demanded to know why my clothes were slovenly and secondhand. It may have been my crooked bangs from the home haircuts, or the burgundy Princeton sweater I wore because it made me feel cool. But it only led to more jests and more jaunts.

* * *

By the time I was in my early twenties, when I was mature enough to recognize the relationship between beauty and commodification, hating my effing face became a full-time obsession. In between modeling and later, stunt jobs, I would literally hide in the mountains, so no one saw my mug. But the years have left their inevitable traces; now that I am no longer beautiful, I can finally admit that I was attractive way back when. I've always regretted that my legs were taken, instead of my face. I could have lived with a scarred, disfigured appearance, but not with these weakened legs. Of course, I had not yet realized the blessings of my relatively intact brain.

After the accident, a couple of nurses at the Dutch spinal cord injury rehabilitation hospital discharged me too early, before I was ready to start my new, disabled life. Maybe I never had been ready. Everywhere I turned seemed a dead end, so after a few years I ventured back to the United States. Originally, I wanted to enroll in a mindfulness program at a Massachusetts hospital, for chronic pain patients. It was organized by Jon Kabat-Zinn, who brought mindfulness meditation to the US. (Jon Kabatt-Zin had also written a book called *Full Catastrophe Living*. I'd loved it, but still went skydiving!)

I was keen to attend the mindfulness classes but wasn't ready to accept that identity or develop an awareness of suffering in my physical shell. I yearned for the *freedom* that came with traveling and roaming, like my heroes Jack Kerouac, Jack London and Martha Geller. After visiting my American best friend Erica—Brooklyn born and bred, from the wrong side of the pre-gentrified tracks—I journeyed by Greyhound, by train, and then as a relocation driver.

Purely by chance, I ended up in Northern Michigan. Maybe meditation at a yoga retreat would help my neurological issues and crushed spirit. *Yes, that'll end well, group meditations for a quirky atheist.* The yoga ranch was based on Paramahansa Yogananda's teachings—I quip on stage I lived in a yoga cult. Two weeks in, I needed to travel back to New York City to pick up my belongings at my best American friend, Erica Obert. My Amtrak pass was still valid, but I was strongly discouraged to leave since "Bad things are going to happen to the Eastern side of the USA." So, like a wuss, I didn't go.

At night, we listened to the cook's cassette player with gloomy, maniacal lectures, "In 2000, forty million people are going to die near the oceans." I didn't fully buy into the cook's Doomsday obsession but did allow groupthink to cloud my common sense. Sadly, I would not see Erica for another decade, and then never again. I left the yoga cult after a few months; the meditations had become mandatory, and I discovered that 'Baba,' the old white guy in charge, slept with his secretary *and* made the moves on another woman. Of course, he told the guy I'd fallen in love with, "Don't associate with Kaatje or you won't ascend." *Yeah, fuck that sexist shit, besides, I already have an old silver haired man in Holland whom I call 'dad.'*

Baba is the East Indian word for 'father,' although in religious and esoteric circles it's also an affectionate name for the head honcho. Baba didn't seem to like it that Eric and I threw dance parties in the domes, or that I had tea parties with girlfriends. Head honchos always desire to rule, and if their followers/underlings start forming strong bonds amongst each other, their power diminishes. There was a lot of fun, too. The others would yell group hug loudly, to give me a heads up so I could run the other way! And of course, I teased Eric mercilessly about inheriting his VCR after he 'ascended.' My departure was therefore bittersweet, as I'd made several close friends.

What I really wanted, to my surprise, was studying. The discipline required distracted me from the post-accident agony, which was slowly worsening. After spending a few happy years at a community college, a mile north of Detroit, the city suddenly did not seem downtrodden enough—and this was before they went broke. I knew of a place that would satisfy my love for more desolate hinterlands than a dying metropolis could offer; a place with mountains, emptiness, and even more hardship. So, I moved to Socorro, New Mexico in the early 2000's. My mom flew in and helped me pack then drive across the country, pulling a 4 x 8 U-Haul trailer behind my little Hyundai hatchback.

That love for junkyards I developed as a child is an essential part of who I am. It's never bothered me to discover half-buried, rusted cars in mesmerizing, bleak landscapes. There's a small trench, part of the Lower Taos Canyon, a few miles south of beautiful Taos, that harbors at least half a dozen cars and trucks. While attending a Writer's Workshop by UNM, I had made my way to the edge of the ravine by using two canes and my leg braces. As usual, fighting with all my might against the physical torment, my left leg and sacrum on fire.

Struggling along, I remembered how, a year after my accident, my parents and I were walking—in my case, limping—around a small lake in the woods near their home. My dad, behind me, jokingly observed, "You're walking the same speed as when you were four years old, on your first mountaineering trip!" *Sure, he was right, and it was also quite typical for him to point out the truth, instead of tactfully saying something like, 'Good job, Kaat!'* My father kept detailed records; receipts, kilometers hiked, altitudes conquered, and children's behavior. Trip journals indicate he was not impressed with my mountaineering skills, at age four: "Very little progress today. Child seems a little uncoordinated and needed a lot of coaxing to keep hiking."

* * *

I still love the wastelands that exists between civilized society and what enabled this life: junkyards, abandoned factories—pretty much everything one can see from an airplane when landing at the Albuquerque International Sunport. Of course, one must know where to look, South Broadway, between Bridge Boulevard and Bobby Foster Road.

Oh New Mexico, you do break my heart sometimes. This is where mobile homes go to die, where people wither away in the harsh desert climate. Hot in the summer, cold in the winter. It always seems windy here, with endless low-blowing clouds of sand carrying tumbleweeds and plastic bags, flying and rolling through the air, only to land, caught, in barbed wire fences. Tumbleweeds, or Russian Thistle, are not native to this area.

Blame the Ukrainian farmers in South Dakota during the late 1800s for spreading the tumbleweed curse across fragile, arid lands; with about 250,000 seeds per plant, they are cruel invaders, killing off native flora. As human immigrants were busy staking out land claims and driving out the native, human population, a tumbleweed crisis probably didn't register as particularly relevant or important at the time.

I cannot fathom how Native Americans and pioneers survived this remote stretch of Planet Earth. New Mexico has an area of 121,697 square miles, or 314,460 square kilometers. The US might have been a slightly saner society, had it used the metric system the Dutch used in Manhattan. American structures would certainly be a lot less crooked. I have yet to meet a framed corner that is exactly 90 degrees. But I digress.

With 17.2 people per square mile, it's empty here, and there's something dreamily romantic about a solitary existence, writing daily in a cabin (I have yet to read *Walden)*. This land has shown me plenty of hardship; yet, brought me happiness. I once owned a lovely little mobile home near Socorro, in the Chihuahuan Desert, that had better insulation and a much higher R-value than the Albuquerque studio I live in now. Lot rent for the mobile home was only $115 a month, and the plot had an unobstructed, 270-degree view of the desert.

Socorro, a beautiful rundown town amidst a background of breathtaking beauty, did not disappoint. Once, I saw a lonesome, grey wolf at the mobile home window, staring at me with piercing eyes. This desert and its wildness reminded me of the books I'd devoured in my youth, *Old Yeller, White Fang, Call of the Wild*, and of course, everything by Mark Twain. I finally had the solitary sanctuary of a little mobile home in the desert, but truly fell in love with a man, and invited him into my life.

* * *

Tall, smart, wonderful Jeremy Jones—my future husband—and I moved in together. Formerly, his name was Jeremy Prasad. Growing up in West-Virginia, children taunted him and called him a "dirty Paki." He took his mother's maiden name, Jones, when he turned eighteen. Jeremy's father was a highly respected Sociology professor, born in Trinidad. Mary, Jeremy's mom, eventually moved back to West-Virginia, after years at a West Coast Ivy League university. Mary raised Jeremy as best as she could as a single mom, but throughout her life carried a tad of hatred toward men, and inevitably, somewhat bullied her son. As a youth, Jeremy could neither raise his voice nor use a hammer, and he was instructed to keep everyone away from the house, as his mom was a fanatical hoarder.

"You are my saucy Hollandaise," Jeremy would tease me, until he realized how many guys I'd been saucy with. I didn't want to hurt him, so I never joked about my tumultuous, pre-accident life, and I certainly did not talk about my NYC, Paris, Tokyo, and Milan modeling days, or other adventures. Bringing that up made him not like me very much, as he was deeply insecure, especially about the guys I'd slept with. As the years wore on, Jeremy became obsessed with my past, and I became obsessed with our present. He was funny, smart, good looking, very kind and he always had female friends who seemed to adore him.

Most annoyingly, they would ask him a little too often for help with their homework or research project. When we met Jeremy was an astrophysics student at New Mexico Tech, where I earned a Psychology degree with a minor in Biology in the early 2000s. I loved the rigor of New Mexico Tech. It was no party school, for even a Bachelor of Science in Psychology required Calc I and II, as well as Calc-based Physics I and II, Intro to Probability, and Programming in C+. There was no grading on a curve either. However, there was student life, and we attended dinners and parties at various homes.

One of Jeremy's best friends was Julia Archuleta, a gorgeous, intelligent blonde with an asshole of a boyfriend. Of course, Julia always confided her sorrows in my then fiancée. One evening, she had invited us and a bunch of other students to their little, stone home near the railroad tracks. Every seat in the place was uncomfortable, despite the blow-up pillow I always carried with me, for my bum. After we finished eating, I had to lie down on their uncomfortable, and quite hard, futon couch, but at least that seemed to alleviate the tailbone anguish a little. From the next room, I heard laughter and muffled voices, and a question floating in the air, "Eh, why is she lying down?"

Sure, I had a cane and leg braces under my long pants and a cane holder on my bicycle, but I probably appeared too normal and healthy to need to lie down at a party. Nonetheless, I had to skip the following semester because of both physical and mental burnout. The pain was a monster, and I recalled how, even a year after my first rehabilitation discharge, I was already schlepping pillows around. Despite what some would guess should have been obvious, I made no connection between the horrifying pain I experienced sitting upright at their dinner table and my skydiving accident. I was as ignorant of my body while at this university as before the skydiving accident.

Lying on their green futon, my thoughts drifted off to childhood, and the last few years. I'd been a smart youth, yet would never describe myself as "precocious," given my spectacular failures. At Oakland Community College's Southfield campus, a Childhood Development class was full of young, black mothers taken the Nursing route. The kind, elderly RN devoted an entire lecture on children who were 'The Golden One' of their families. These children needed extra protection from predators, especially in their early teens. I loved that class, there was such a sense of unity and cohesion, perhaps because all of us were profoundly motivated to escape our circumstances.

For me, that meant avoiding any job that would require prolonged standing. Because I had underperformed academically for most of my life, I didn't even see there were options for me like a job in HR, law or research, despite earning straight A's. *Maybe I can become a Paramedic, so I won't have to work in McDonalds for the rest of my life.* In the computer lab, another black classmate scoffed at my dreams of becoming a Paramedic. She said it was *blue-collar*, that she personally wouldn't stop till she was a neuro-surgeon. Smart girl.

* * *

That first semester at New Mexico Tech, weeks after meeting the love of my life, I fell violently ill in the middle of finals. I had severe leg spasms, which I now understand, were triggered by a 105-degree fever irritating the old, incomplete spinal cord damage and the cauda equina syndrome. It felt like my head was exploding; there was a pounding sensation in the back of my neck. I was nauseated and shivered from head to toe, and light hurt my eyes. I ended up in the ER, and a butcher of a small-town physician insisted on a spinal tap—otherwise known as a lumbar puncture. A head CT had already shown a raging sinus infection, and a kind nurse whispered to me, "You don't need to do anything you don't want to, you know?"

Because I had a 105-degree fever, and there were concerns about an infection in my spinal cord or brain, it felt I had no choice. I told the doctor to be careful because of the sacral and lumbar nerve damage from the sky diving accident. The moment the needle went in, I yelled for her to pull it out; it felt as if my left leg was suddenly amputated. An overwhelming, sharp, shooting and stabbing sensation from my waist to my left foot ensued. I screamed and screamed while she just kept going, telling me to lie quietly. It seems unimaginable, but the torment from the lumbar puncture had been more painful than landing at 70 mph, obliterating sacral nerves.

In retrospect, I can't help but wonder how many patients with chronic pain have had similar encounters: as a result of this unnecessary medical test, I sustained another injury to the cauda equina plexus, and I am pretty confident she pierced a nerve or two. A course of antibiotics soon cleared up bacterial sinusitis, but I was unaware that I might never recover from that lumbar puncture. I shrugged off the residual, sharp left leg pain and continued an exhausting race with myself and my body to obtain my degree so I could apply to Physician Assistant schools. I was oblivious to the fact the race was rigged, and a strange sounding disease would befall me.

* * *

As for Jeremy and me, well, we built a good life together, for a while. I've always been an avid do-it-yourselfer (DIY), but my dad did not have the patience to teach me, so learned everything myself as a Dutch teenager and young homeowner. Being self-taught was much harder, and I made plenty of mistakes when I bought my first fixer-upper at age 22. I succeeded only because I inherited my father's spectacular DIY abilities, along with his tenacity for completing hard projects.

Although neither Jeremy nor I had been taught how to fix things, in my upbringing creativity was greatly encouraged, even expected. From crafting wooden, temporary shacks from sticks and scraps to drawing and painting, I cannot remember my parents holding us back. Whereas Jeremy, an incredibly hard worker, wasn't even allowed to use a hammer as a child or teen, and later on would procrastinate on turning in a work assignment, or a simple Ikea assembly. What complicated matters was that Jeremy had a hard time organizing projects, even if he excelled at computers and math.

Sure, I was a master at home improvement but lacked the physical strength to carry out all my brilliant schemes, and that gave rise to great frustration, for both of us. For our first home together in Albuquerque, I'd wanted a low key, modern townhome with level floors, while Jeremy wanted the dream of a single-family home although he had never gardened or owned a home before. I loathed our badly insulated, 1950's home from the moment we moved in, as it required more maintenance than I had the energy for.

Despite our efforts, the real homewrecker, adhesive arachnoiditis, lurked in the shadows, out of sight. I blamed my physical agony for the demise of my marriage, but of course there were other factors. Attributing the pain to my 2009 divorce may be a logical fallacy called *post hoc ergo propter hoc*, which is Latin for *after this, therefore because of this*. The post hoc fallacy happens when we erroneously assume that because one thing occurred after another thing, the second thing happened as a result of the first.

In my view, we justify our actions after our brains have already made the decision. From buying a home, to choosing whom to marry—or divorce, to stealing a bonbon at the Borders bookstore checkout counter ("It looked like it was free," my friend will defend her actions to this day), everything humanity does, including writing this book, is done under post hoc reasoning. In other words, we can ponder, and our brains feed off our delusions, but it won't really matter.

* * *

Over my life I've made so many logical fallacies when it comes to decision making. Sadly, never once have I prioritized my health. When I feel really, really sorry for myself, which does not happen often, this is one of my favorite lamenting fantasies: *Should have stayed in Detroit and attended Wayne State, where I'd already scouted a cute, 350 square foot, rundown studio on the eleventh floor, in 1999.* The apartment was right across from the University, and at that time, I could have limped to class just fine. Detroit was also a one-way flight to and from Amsterdam, which would have made it much easier to fly home to visit the family.

If I had stayed in Detroit, I never would have suffered a lumbar puncture injury which most certainly sealed my fate as a bedridden patient in the decades to come. If I had stayed in Detroit, I never would have met, married, and divorced Jeremy, one of the saddest losses I've ever known. I wanted to be more than just my disability; more than someone who suffered nerve, spine and musculoskeletal damage. I wanted to have a life and a meaningful job and figured that was best accomplished by leaving Michigan forever. The sad fact is, some people cannot outrun, or limp, from their inner hinterlands, no matter how hard they try.

PART TWO

My day job, modeling in Paris

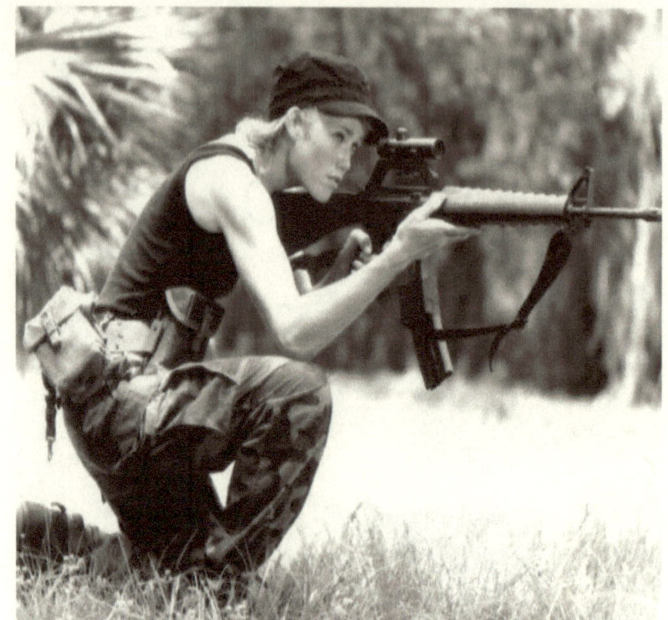

Florida stuntschool, afterwards was hired for a Dutch movie and two TV shows.
Conquering the 3905 meter Ortler Mtn.

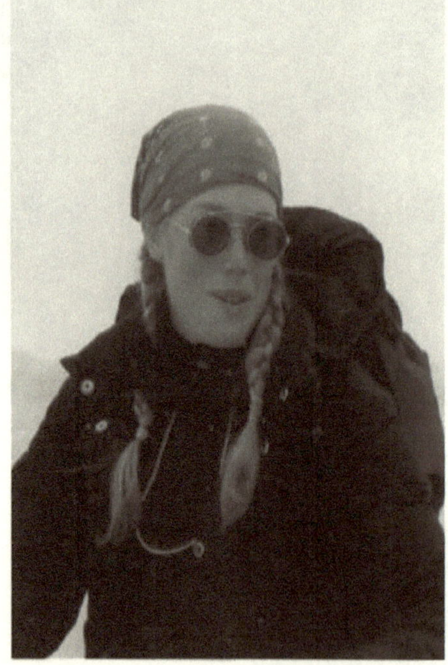

Loving my first job as a PA-C, in Gastroenterology.

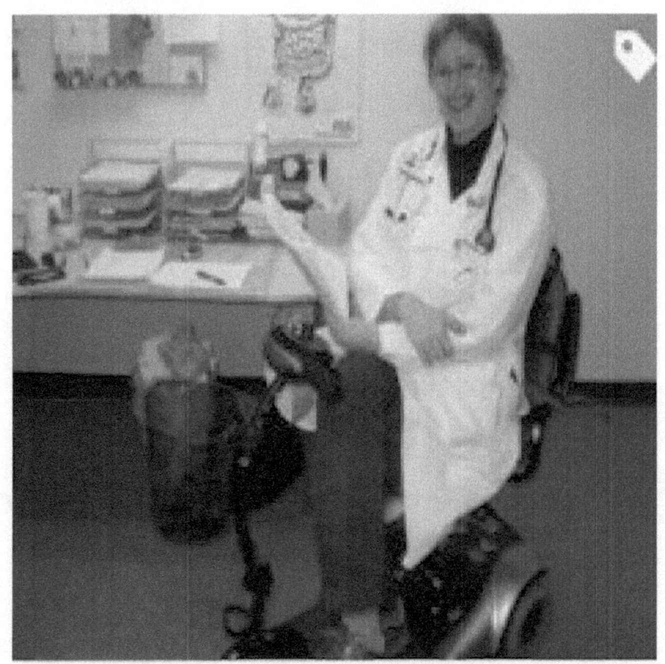

Definitely not loving my day job; magazine covers from Tokyo, Paris, Milan and Belgium.

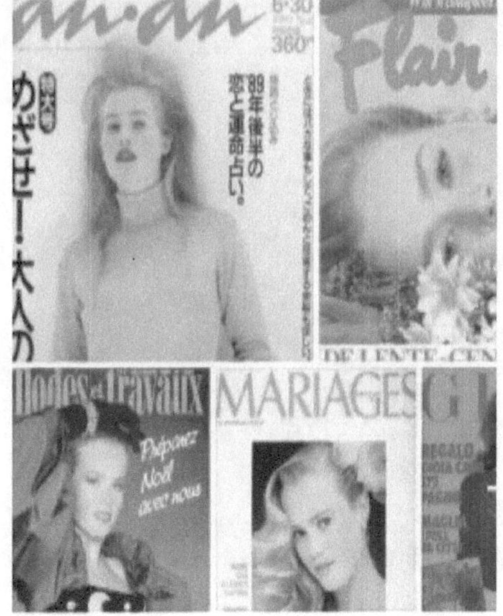

3 SOLIPSISM SYNDROME, OR BUST!*

To label any subject unsuitable for comedy is to admit defeat. Sometimes reality is so horrible we refuse to face it unless trapped by comedy. - Peter Sellers

I'm in yet another doctor's office, trying to find a Primary Care provider that is closer than Meadowlark Family Healthcare, a 35-minute drive. I did not like this Presbyterian provider's attitude. While he's running me through the standard questionnaire, twice his medical assistants shoved an Opioid Contract under my nose. I wasn't even there for an opioid prescription, and he'd already refused to prescribe an intranasal ketamine spray. He'd never heard of severe, residual pain from crushed, damaged sacral nerves and wasn't interested to learn more.

"Do you ever have fleeting suicidal thoughts?" he finally asked, seemingly exasperated.

"Eh....no."

I'd learned to lie aloud to nurses, health care providers or therapists, while silently thinking, *Nope, they are not fleeting, they're pretty fucking persistent.* Another provider would ask, "Do you have passive suicidal thoughts, like if you get hit by a truck and died, it will not matter?"

"No, not really," I'd answer while contemplating, *I am an atheist, so of course it would not matter. With my luck though, I'd survive and end up with a complete quadriplegic injury, on a ventilator or sustain an amputation or two. I know the way the cookie crumbles.*

I feared that one of two things would happen if I told a medical provider how severe my physical torment was, or about how I wished for a quick death: either they would take away medications because they'd consider me a potential overdose candidate, or they would refer me to some sort of in-patient psychiatric treatment program. Where certainly, they'd attribute my moans a psych issue while refusing to provide pain medications. It's the dilemma for chronic pain patients, everywhere. If we're honest, it will make life even more difficult to bear.

But I knew all their tricks, from my own years in Primary Care, Psychiatry and Urgent Care. My suicidal thoughts may not have been fleeting, but I refused to feel depressed; I knew I always had a way out, if necessary. I have a lot of meds that, if taken all at once, would certainly relieve me of my physical anguish. When a person is in dire enough circumstance but not ready to end it all, it is a comfort to know one can check out. And it's a logical conclusion, devoid of suicidal feelings: why should I continue, prevail in this body, with these hardships?

Amitriptyline, a tricyclic antidepressant and one of my prescribed neuropathic pain medications, is super effective. An overdose guarantees liver failure, and they'd never get me on a donor list in time. I'd just have to hide the bottle, so they wouldn't know what I took. That plan's problem is, if I made it far enough to progress to unconsciousness, and I was taken to a hospital, they'd run a basic blood test and find elevated liver enzymes, and they'd figure it out quickly.

Of course, my medication list is in most computerized systems, and one look at my yellow-tinged skin would signal liver failure to the paramedics. What's one way to do it they couldn't detect? I could stop eating and drinking fluids. It only takes about ten days, and it is painless, according to the website *Death with Dignity*.[39] Unless, of course, someone discovers I'm in trouble and they take me to the hospital, as my Advanced Directives are not signed yet. What is that about?

* * *

My fantastic therapist, Hope, like the half dozen before her in Holland, the UK, and the US, diagnosed me with situational depression. It sounds innocuous, as if the depression would resolve if my situation was different and my spinal cord injuries and inflammation were gone. In my case, situational depression seems even more damning than a diagnosis of major depression. Because my situation, in many ways, deteriorated over time.

I've been a prisoner of increasing, physical torture for over twenty years. Each year has brought more agony than the one before, so my grief has never been complete. The accident happened in 1992, and aside from the one-year spinal cord rehabilitation in 1992/1993, I had rehabbed as an outpatient in 1994, 2003, and as an inpatient again in 2015. Every decade, heck, every year, I've had to say goodbye to more and more "normal" functioning of my body.

I'm in bed twenty-two, if not twenty-three, hours a day. I write on a laptop, my body turned to the right side, a pillow propping me up on both sides. As always, I have an icepack pressed against my sacrum. It helps trick my brain into ignoring the internal burning sensations. Often, it's becoming harder and harder to fall asleep, and not just from the PTSD. I will doze off, only to jerk awake seconds later, in terror and disbelief. *Me! In bed for most of the rest of my life.* I wake up clawing at my chest, telling my body to calm down. It feels as if my heart is throwing up in my rib cage, my body violently purging the loathing I feel for my life. Somehow, I know that I will never get used to the solitary confinement.

Lying in a fetal position on my right side is the only way to cope because any pressure on the sacrum worsens the neuropathic pain. Lying directly on my back, even on a memory foam mattress, causes excruciating torment after only twenty or thirty minutes. I can't even write for more than forty-five minutes at a time. My sacrum cannot bear the weight of me—in any position. The gnawing sacral pain and left leg agony are bad enough, but lately, it feels as if a vizor is wrapped around the base of my skull and there is a pounding, buzzing sensation in the back of my neck.

The most minute chore, like making a sandwich, causes my body to react like there's a switch in my brain that terminates my central nervous system; I literally pass out for a few hours. The nerve pain itself is a burning, electrical sensation traveling from my chest all the way down to my toes. Everything seems to exacerbate it. Moving around. Going to the restroom. Prepping a meal. The clothes on my skin. The cold air from the fridge. Ceiling fans. Being alive hurts every single second. And then I remembered. In Riverside General, they'd provided a bed tunnel for my feet.

The weight of the sheets and hospital blankets intensified the searing, burning sensations, so a metal cage was placed in bed, to free my lower legs. I was years away from understanding neurological ache, how the skin of my legs, buttocks, and feet could feel so numb and cold yet simultaneously hurt that much on the inside. The skin on my buttocks, back of my legs, vulva, clitoris and perineum including the anus, has been completely numb on the left since the accident. The right side used to have a little feeling, although that is diminishing too.

* * *

By the summer of 2015, my ache had reached around a daily eight to nine —a ten is my skydiving accident—and nothing seemed to diminish the pain levels. Life was no longer worth living. I needed to know why I was hurting this much, and most importantly, why it was still increasing. The uncertainty was driving me to despair. I made an appointment with New Mexico Orthopedics, not expecting much.

Most orthopedic medical providers are not known for their empathy and compassion, but my spine doctor looked sad and teary eyed. Dr. Cheng patiently explained that the gnawing and burning pain I experienced originated from *lumbosacral adhesive arachnoiditis*. It hit me then, from my medical education and working in Spinal Cord Injuries, that meningeal inflammation and scar tissue meant a life lost, a body destroyed…all that hard work of the last twenty years for naught.

"There is nothing medicine can do for you. I'm deeply sorry."

"I don't understand. What kind of life will I have to lead, Dr. Cheng? What are my options?" I mumbled, feeling my tears well up like water behind a badly maintained 1930s WPA dam, ready to burst.

"Well, obviously, a very quiet and calm life," he replied.

Oh no he didn't. After the verdict, I cried. I hated crying because sobbing always worsened my sacral and trunk agony. Even regular breathing worsened the sharp, burning discomfort from my left sided chest, abdomen and back. I left Dr Cheng's office and limped behind my walker back to my previous minivan. It was parked in a scorching hot, black asphalt lot, a shimmering sea mirage in the New Mexico summer heat. I immediately called my mom.

"Why hadn't anyone," I cried, "…any of the doctors I'd seen, explained this to me?" Various medical providers had given me bits and pieces of my larger pain syndrome diagnosis puzzle, but this was the first time a doctor had connected all the dots. What I saw as new symptoms in 2015 was exactly what I'd felt in 2005. It came as quite a shock to finally have a more comprehensive, meaningful diagnosis, and with that diagnosis, I learned my prognosis was grim.

Lumbosacral adhesive arachnoiditis, Tarlov cysts and *thecal sac abnormalities* had shown up on every MRI taken since the mid-2000s. In 2005, a thoracic lesion was discovered by Dutch Neurologist Dr. Vos, who did an actual physical examination, a rarity these days. Dr. Vos applied a tuning fork and rubber hammer to numerous areas of my body, he tested all my dermatomes with a piece of cotton and a sharp paperclip. Soon, Dr. Vos notified me I had lost all my upper and lower motor reflexes as well as anal sphincter tone. Yup, he was thorough!

This brilliant Dutch diagnostician didn't need MRIs, just a thorough, standardized American Spinal Injury Association (ASIA) neurology exam to determine the exact location of my third spinal cord/spinal cord root injury. I was told that the T4 spinal cord lesion, most likely, happened from shearing forces sustained during the sky diving accident.

Despite having these various diagnoses—Brown-Sequard, cauda equina syndrome, T4 lesion—no one had ever painted the whole neuropathic picture, and they never spelled out what it meant for my future. At the time, I did some of my own research and read that Brown-Sequard usually went away, so I didn't connect that 2005 diagnosis with my current, severe left-sided trunk pain. It also helps to be in denial, doesn't it?

* * *

After the visit with Dr. Cheng, I literally crawled back into bed and grabbed the only notebook I had, a *free* gift from that overpriced, but helpful Master Workshop at the UNM Taos Writer's Conference in 2014. The hotel was a nightmare for mobility impaired people, but I was still eager and excited, and ventured to the welcome hall with my two-wheel mobility scooter, leg braces and cane. After seeing the long line for the badges, and without a comfortable seat on the spiffy scooter, I asked for help from one of the welcoming committee, a longhaired, turquoise dripping older female. Uh-oh. Legs buckling, I kneeled to the tiled ground, asked for a chair to sit on and explained; "I have spinal cord damage and am in a lot of pain."

"Sure," she replied, "but I can't give you special treatment, you'll still have to wait in line." Sheesh, I know her type, didn't expect special treatment anyway. I was forced to drag the metal chair along, the snake-like line moving slowly against the orange and peach Taos sunset. Schlepping a cane and a backpack on my little scooter meant I didn't have an extra pair of hands for a pillow, so I sat uncomfortably on my right leg to avoid my tailbone and buttocks touching the metal surface.

The volunteer could have easily helped, but this was quintessential UNM behavior, I didn't even question it. I just *sensed* that people like her appeared caring and warm, yet it was a facade of kindness, an empty mirage. Whether they smelled of patchouli, deodorant or Clinique's Happy eau de parfum;

nothing could have masked the smell of their hollow, rotting hearts. I didn't even have the vocabulary to identify what just happened, still blissfully unaware of the word *ableist*, despite 26 months of UNM education.

Previously I'd attended St. Francis Physician Assistant school, after Jeremy and I escaped from Connecticut. Unfortunately, St. Francis didn't offer cadaver dissection, and Dr. A., one of the professors seemed a creepy ignoramus. This man had a Ph.D. in Exercise Science, but his main qualifications were teaching remedial Gross Anatomy to medical students who'd failed their exams. Many an Anatomy session consisted of drawing muscles on each other with dry erasers, while wearing shorts and an exercise bra.

Dr. A. wanted to "help" by touching my inner groin, to demonstrate the exact location of the adductor longus. My entire left leg up to my waist was on fire and hurting badly that day, but I also didn't want his hands there, at all. For once in my life, I made my boundaries known, so when he said, "Do I have your permission to palpate the muscle insertion point?" I friendly and firmly answered, "No." A bright red, raging Dr. A. immediately banned me to the hallway, shortly afterwards I was disciplined and threatened by the PA Director and his VP. What a clusterfuck of a situation.

A few months ago, in the beginning of our PA education, one day I excitedly, and innocently hollered; "Yes, isn't it amazing, we *are* related to apes" to which Dr. A. had replied, while glaring at me angrily: "That's only if you believe in those balderdash theories!" Since Professor A. was also responsible for grading our Master thesis project, I had little faith he would judge me fairly. Classic example of a sunk cost fallacy; keep going since I'd already invested so much time and money, or spend another year and a half miserable and stressed?

After the exceptional education at Quinnipiac University, New Mexico Tech, and Oakland Community College, a mile North of Detroit's Eight Mile Road, these new experiences left me in shock. I assumed a public university would have an excellent ADA policy in place. Before transferring to the UNM PA Program though, I'd met with a professional disability coordinator at UNM's South Campus. She was passionate yet pragmatic, and throughout my PA education her department assisted by cutting up my 15 lbs., 2500-page textbooks into smaller, portable parts. But for the bulk of the didactic part, I was at the mercy of UNM North, since that's where the PA school was located.

Astonishingly, UNM North's disability counselor was a platitude spouting hippie, all feely goody without any common sense. This counselor seemed incapable of coming up with disability solutions, so I brought in padded chairs for lectures, and a thickly cushioned Costco shop stool for the cadaver lab myself. Unbelievably, she once taught a medical school lecture—to foster empathy and creativity—by asking us to imagine *You're a tree, blowing in the wind.*

Ultimately it was the head librarian and blue-collar workers who would get me through PA school. The librarian provided access to a tiny, private room/closet where I stored my mat and sleeping bag so I could rest my spine over lunch. Additionally, the blue-collar heroes from the medical school's basement came up with practical solutions such as storing my scooter in an engine room, to which they cut me a key. I still had to arrive an hour early, because the handicap spots closest to the engine room were quickly taken by able bodied folks, medical students among them—I kid you not.

I'd hoped to park the mobility scooter at the PA School hallway, which was closer to mostly unused accessible parking spots. In tears, I had shown my primary care physician's letter, requesting help for my disability, to no avail. While I was limping with leg braces and a cane, one punk-ass student went joyriding on my scooter despite my protests, another insisted my wheelchair couldn't be in a group photo, and another taunted, "Hey, why don't you join our weekly runner's group?"

Perhaps I seemed an enigma—my upper body strength, stuntwoman background and faith in ropes and carabiners meant I'd ruled the "Team Building" challenge course in orientation week, which did not require any walking or standing. Literally, the only physical activity I excelled at, aside from swimming, was a small obstacle course relying on my upper body strength.

There was little to no support for medical and PA students with physical challenges; another disabled medical student had to withdraw from the program after the intense Gross Anatomy summer semester, and I was 'on my own' once again.

Sadly, the undue physical stress surely influenced my outlook negatively and hampered my learning. I attended the intense morning medical school lectures, rested over lunch at the library, made it through the afternoon PA school lectures and practicals, rushed home with a weary spine, and spend the rest of the evening studying in a second hand Lazy-Boy.

During the first year, one of the senior professors cornered me over and over. He'd accost me in hallways, or while waiting for the elevator, demanding to know why my grades were average instead of commensurate with my intelligence. I lacked the energy, and trust, to tell him about my struggles and was annoyed at his persistence. Sure, the lack of support for my disability isolated me, but my own attitude and comparison to New Mexico Tech, did me no favors ("I can't believe UNM grades on a curve!").

I seemed to survive by latching onto to glimpses of kindness wherever I could find it; the head of the Gross Anatomy lab, an inspiring PA or medical school lecturer, a professor with CRPS, a visiting, excellent embryology lecturer, a bookstore employee, wonderful, smart PA preceptors and a couple of outstanding, medical and PA students.

By the time I graduated in 2008, my marriage had deteriorated steadily under the strain until finally our beautiful love blew away across the New Mexico landscape like those tumbleweeds, the Russian Thistle. Meanwhile, a brand-new Pete Domenici Center had been built for the medical school and modern cadaver lab. Once again, UNM hadn't even allocated $2000 for a handicap button to operate the heavy door to the accessible bathroom—and the women's breastfeeding station. Yet across from that inaccessible bathroom, $100,000 artwork was on display. Didn't they know that pretty paintings do not magically open bathroom doors? I swear it looked as if it was intentionally designed by that North Campus disability coordinator. There was no other explanation, for a building that would end up costing $600 million.

For the most part though, without study groups or note sharing, I did Physician Assistant school alone. That isn't a good coping strategy, but I'd read too much Jack London, had solo-hiked and climbed too many mountains not to rely on rugged individualism. Besides, I was extremely motivated to contribute to society as a PA. It wasn't UNM's fault that socially, I'd only ever thrived in tightknit skydiving and mountaineering communities. But I fell in love with medicine, and most of all, getting to know and help people from different backgrounds within a collaborative provider-patient relationship. Whereas my team failed me over and over, my diligence, candidness and humor seemed not only appreciated but welcomed by patients.

* * *

Never mind all that, let's get back to my current crisis. My orthopedic physician had diagnosed me with 'adhesive arachnoiditis,' and I quit crying long enough to open a bag of neon sour gummi worms to start writing what would be my first stand-up comedy joke. My precious Pepper, the rescue Siamese/Calico kitten that my ex and I had adopted in Socorro, was purring on my bed. Pepper lived with me in hotels when I worked as a locum tenens PA, she traveled back and forth across the Atlantic Ocean, but she was happiest right here with me, at home.

I could not stop writing comedy and will never stop. My first comedy notes read, "Oh Oprah. I do hold you responsible for unleashing all evil in the world, like Dr. Phil and Dr. Oz. Screw Oprah, and the medical, and scientific, ignorance she propagated. And, yeah, fuck those gratitude journals." Given that I could no longer feel grateful about anything in my life, that became my new daily mantra. Too many people rely on the power of positive thinking to overcome the insurmountable, but sometimes, that is simply not enough.

I'm scolding you, Louisa L. Hay! Believing that we are deficient because we cannot think our way out of our physical torment, poverty or poor health, is merely another form of self-punishment and is not psychologically healthy. Famous Dutch author, disability advocate and essayist Karin Spaink, calls this travesty the *oren mafia* aka Ear Mafia, or as she relayed via personal communication; "The best English translation is *Mob Mind*." In my case, going in the opposite direction became a saving grace, and my first stage joke about Oprah would be a thing that pulled me through.

In the spring and summer of 2015, I had been working part-time for Dr. Gingery, a smart, wonderful Geriatric Psychiatrist. I'd even done my Physician Assistant elective rotation in Psychiatry, so I finally felt as if I landed my dream job. But the Nursing Home where I provided consults and care had long, thick, carpeted hallways. While I went from room to room, that carpet became my enemy. It would greet me in the morning, at which point I had to choose how I would move around that day. I could either use my walker and leg braces, or I could use my manual wheelchair.

Both options seemed to increase the severity of my suffering. Outside observers of people who need assistive devices underestimate the difficulties associated with not being able to move like a person without physical challenges. Walking unevenly or compensating /adjusting the body to avoid pain is a hazard for many, because it leads to inflammation and dysfunction in otherwise healthy parts of the body. What *seems* accessible to the abled-bodied usually isn't.

Independently owned coffeeshops may use a hallway to store jute bags of coffee, blocking the path to the large, accessible toilet. This is just one example, but you get the picture. This doesn't just affect me, it concerns the aging, the deaf community, the visually impaired; the US is not prioritizing the upcoming tsunami of an aging population with disability needs. At least not the way they strategize and implement public policy in South Korea, or Japan.

* * *

Furthermore, my original disability aggravated my ankle joints and feet. Years of overusing my legs, pushing my body when I should have been resting, and landing more on the left side during the accident, meant an abnormal, uneven gait. My leg braces, cane, and a walker could not fully prevent limping, or that waddling walk of mine, called a 'Trendelenburg gait.' My lack of proprioception—knowing where one's limbs are in whatever position—made it worse. My left foot had been weaker, more atrophied than the right since the accident, and the ligaments were lax.

The more I walked, basically anything over 100 feet, or was upright *too much* my left ankle joint would swell, it looked as if there was an egg just below the ankle bone. I had never regained the ability to push off or stand on my toes, which meant walking on my heels which led to undue pressure on the weakened ankle joints. I developed pressure sores from my leg braces, which needed constant tending. Since 2013, 2014, after every shift, I'd crawl in bed with one ice pack on my sacrum and one on my left ankle. The icepacks stayed there until I had to work again.

I forced my body and did not want to give up my life as a professional, not when it gave me so much joy, and finally being really good at something. As the years passed, mustering the mental energy to walk behind a walker or with a cane became too exhausting. My mind had to think about every step, and that was extremely tiring. So, I often opted for the wheelchair. It had the additional benefit of allowing me to carry four or five paper charts in my lap at a time. Of course, the weight of the files stacked on my sensitive, aching legs severely worsened the sacral ache, with my low back pressed against the chair.

With every oscillation, propelling myself forward, I greatly agitated my sacrum by creating more pressure against the backrest. The thick carpet underneath the wheels made it quite difficult to gather any momentum. The longer I was sitting upright, the more the trunk, chest and especially sacral affliction intensified. This was aggravated by my shortened trunk. Since I lost two inches of spinal height during the accident, the rib cage was much closer to my hipbones, and it rubbed against the ileac crest. That gave rise to even more discomfort, and nociceptive—tissue—pain.

While I was heartbroken over it, I had to give up work, and shortly afterwards the Federal government awarded disability at the first try. At the time, I was still hopeful I could return part-time, and blamed it all on the carpet. But of course, it was due to the severity of combined pain syndromes. As for life outside of work, I had to face the fact that I lost most of my mobility that year so began using the wheelchair daily. The sacral, leg and foot aching had such a burning quality to it, I could no longer sit, stand, or walk, even for a few minutes. When I moved about the house, I crawled until finally, I needed to spend even more hours in bed.

On my last day at the Nursing Home I decided to give my spiffy Dutch walker to a vet with diabetic neuropathy and alcohol use disorder. He had one of those ridiculous American walkers, where the physical therapist slices a couple of tennis balls and places them over the legs so the walker glides. Bizarrely, his generic walker looked like it came from a Russian cold war depot, yet cost the same as my wonderful, sleek—and more functional— European walker. I didn't regret giving the walker away because my legs had never felt worse, and I wanted to do something nice for the ailing vet.

* * *

Days turned into weeks, and I kept writing comedy in bed, in total isolation until one afternoon, an old friend invited me out, to celebrate his engagement. I forced my lonely, aching body to Marble Brewing's patio to meet my good British/Italian friend Derek and his wonderful fiancé. I'd met Derek at a regional Burning Man event where I was on medical duty earlier that year. Out of loneliness, in 2014 and 2015 I'd attended EDM—electronic dance music—concerts, the regional Burning Man, and even a Phish concert —turns out I hate Phish, and Phish fans, even more. Overall, I enjoyed EDM, the culture and meeting new people but hadn't realized I'd still end up feeling like the sober outcast.

Marble Brewing was noisy, I suffered more for going out, but had fun for the first time in weeks. Derek's friend Marty Adam Smith seemed nice, we shared a chat and a laugh. I confided I'd written some comedy stuff, although I heavily guarded the fact my jokes were written from bed. I did not want to seem lazy and hadn't even told Derek about my deteriorating situation yet.

"So, what is it about comedy that interests you?" Marty asked, himself an improv performer and comedian. "Really, comedy is the last vestige of a civilized society, before total collapse is imminent," I replied eagerly, not knowing some was unconsciously picked up from Bill Hicks, whose comedy I had yet to see. Or perhaps it was parallel thinking. Because Bill Hicks actually had said, "Comedy is the last bastion of free speech."

Marty told me to keep writing, then laughed encouragingly, "It sounds like you need to go to an open mic and get started." Marty helped me limp back to my wheelchair, twenty feet further. The adrenaline of being outside my bed must have worn off, because abruptly the Marble Brewing vibe felt tiresome and loud. My nostrils and acute sense of smell inevitably were attacked by the aroma of a baby boomer's ass-sweat soaked leather pants, beers that were too strong, and the occasional whiff of gas. Delicious humanity, when you're sitting in your wheelchair, nose at genital level during a Grateful Dead tribute band.

I was too petrified to perform the jokes I had written, at an open mic. However, I knew David Garcia, a musician who ran a mixed open mic—with comedy and music—at a pub nearby. Best of all, "The Draft Station" had a couch for me to lie on. A few months earlier I'd mustered up the courage to read the intro to a previous, now abandoned memoir. Danny Danger's gentle guitar music had accompanied me, because I could not yet face an audience alone, with my soft, insecure voice and Dutch accent.

* * *

When I grabbed the mic for the first time on August 18, 2015, like most comics I had three goals: *get laughter, get a beer, and get laid.* Eventually, by those standards I would become a stellar success. I was in an inordinate amount of anguish yet managed to drag my smarting body out of bed and make it to the Draft Station's open mic night, every Tuesday. It was far from easy. It required careful planning, such as a hot bath with Epsom Salt beforehand and bringing a blanket and Hot Toes.

I began to rely more and more on comedy that reflected my misery while making fun of my disease which turned out to be 'adhesive arachnoiditis.' My favorite: "Fuck. I wish I was normal and had fibromyalgia!" Of course, that is an agonizing condition, but seems a tad more treatable than adhesive arachnoiditis. Besides, it's just a silly joke, I wouldn't want to wish fibromyalgia on anyone. Although medical research indicates that healthy food, gentle exercise, and maintaining a stable weight go a long way when it comes to chronic pain; neuropathy—and perhaps fibromyalgia too—is much harder to treat.

On stage, I embellished the truth, joking that my handsome, Asian-American spine doc had said: "'Well, the bad news is that you suffer from bone cancer like pain. The good news is…you won't die.' So naturally, I started smoking the next day. I needed an exit strategy, stat! Fuck me over triple sideways though, smoking isn't a guarantee, only 1/3 are environmentally linked." In reality, a few weeks ago Dr Cheng had explained mine was one of the most serious, most tormenting conditions. Since he'd given me the diagnosis with moist, sad eyes—and orthopedic providers were known for no nonsense bedside manners—I sensed how hopeless it was, this 'adhesive arachnoiditis.' Yet I yearned for my notebook to come alive in front of an audience.

And yet. And yet. It is hard to convey the suffering from adhesive arachnoiditis without grasping for concepts such as *bone cancer like pain*. But that's exactly what the sacrum and low back feel like, as if it is being destroyed by malignant cells. Of course, the nerves and nerve roots, directly underneath the spinal cord, *are* being annihilated, by inflammation and scar tissue. After reading that I closed my Googling on the topic for over a year. I didn't want to know.

* * *

I continued swimming and physical therapy exercises religiously, including stretches three to four times a week, even when my body screamed to keep lying horizontally, in fetal position. Although for the last 15 years, swimming always made me feel a little better, I could neither outswim the pain nor my situation. Regular depression, and chronic physical agony, may be alleviated with Cognitive Behavioral Therapy (CBT), exercise, and walks in nature. Where were my fucking walks in nature? *Situational depression, indeed.*

Come to think of it, comedy is the only art form that allowed me to become an adult, to set free that crushed and bullied child within. Keeping myself upright, even in the wheelchair, wasn't easy as I couldn't focus as much on delivery of my jokes. The physical discomfort seriously interfered, but it was too late. I was hooked, and soon, other hosts asked me to join their comedy-only open mics. While I wrote new comedy material and kept going to open mics, now twice a week, life went on for my family overseas, too.

My father's Alzheimer's worsened, my Dutch mobile home needed to be cleaned out and I was homesick. So, in the Fall of 2015 I made the arduous journey home, before Henk had forgotten my existence. The 18-hour trip back and forth greatly aggravated the adhesive arachnoiditis, shortly after my return flight I was hospitalized at Lovelace. Since their resident Physical Therapist/wheelchair expert had determined I could sit nor stand nor walk properly, she had me try out a power wheelchair. When I rode around, for the first time ever in a power wheelchair, I cried and said, "If I had had one of these going through PA school and work, that would have saved my marriage."

It hit me hard, the realization that solutions such as an electrical hospital bed, power wheelchair and home health would have meant I could have made my life, and marriage, work. The upside of Lovelace was the support by my friend Meredith, another disabled medical provider, we were hospitalized at the same time. Meredith—a Nurse Practitioner—understood what it was like, being a medical provider banned to the other side of health care. We visited each other's rooms all the time, it was incredulous that both of us had gone boating with our friend Deb Grady two years earlier. I'd even crawled on hands and feet, atop a large rock and had thrown my body into Lake Abiquiu. Meredith and I had been relentless, an invincible team on the inflatable while Deb raced her speed boat faster and faster, spinning us out of control.

One week after the Lovelace rehabilitation discharge, my beloved 15-year-old cat Pepper died. It was the only living thing my ex-husband and I had shared, the last reminder of our married life. I'd found her at the New Mexico Tech Physics Department's parking lot in the winter of 2000, shivering and hungry she'd jumped in my car. Heartbroken, I honored Pepper by doing an outrageously funny set on Steven Seagal, weed and terrorists that evening.

* * *

Nevertheless, my persistent thoughts of suicide did not win out. I realized that, if I leave now, there's no way to know how the story ends. I asked myself: *What's going to happen next year, or the year after that?* As I had for ten years prior, I promised myself one more year, even though the agony worsened, my life sucked, and I saw no way out. Somehow, during that year, the pendulum swung in favor of a choice—to remain in the land of the living —as it had every year over the past decade.

My life seemed a puzzle I hadn't fully solved yet, and I embraced the year 2016 by realizing it'd be silly to leave now, without knowing the answer. But comedy itself provided a tiny sprout of hope, and I cherished the time spend outside my hospital bed. Equally important, there remains comfort in knowing I can check out at any time, something I do not confess to family, friends or health care providers.

I often ask myself whether this life is worth it. I'm just a little spark of consciousness, housed in a defunct body, careening toward a downward death spiral. Of course, like all of us are. In my *situation* though, it seems more than reasonable to go to sleep, only to never wake up again. However, slowly but surely, I started to like being me. This was a real feat, given that I'd spent decades disliking myself.

At first, I couldn't figure out what changed. I just knew that laughs profoundly sustained me. Doing stand-up was a thrill, much like skydiving but with a working parachute. It was fun, knowing that this time, gravity would not kill me.

"Hey," I started my sets, "be honest. Does this wheelchair make me look…fat?"

* Wikipedia features the most suitable definition: Solipsism syndrome refers to a psychological state in which a person feels that reality is not external to his or her mind. Periods of extended isolation may predispose people to this condition. (The addition of 'Or Bust!' is my homage to physicist Dr. Richard Feynman and his extraordinary, lifelong curiosity, described in *Tuva or Bust!*)

4. WELCOME TO HELL

"I'm just a survivor from the train wreck of the modern world." - Known to Evil, by Walter Mosley

A ge seventeen, I'd moved to Paris after failing three school years in a row. I always attributed that to loathing school, perhaps it was another case of *post hoc* fallacy. But it seemed pointless, after Caroline passed away the day before her fifteenth birthday—the last of our Scouting friends to die. I felt so forlorn, lonely, and heartbroken, even more so when my first boyfriend broke up with me, weeks after Caroline's death. Staying in Holland no longer seemed an option, but first, I traveled to the UK by myself for her funeral, with only the epic *Mushashi* tome for company.

Two and a half years earlier, age fourteen, I'd taken this same Hoek van Holland-Harwich ferry to celebrate Christmas with Edward and Caroline's family. Rosy, their beloved Labrador was still alive, and we had hiked across misty fields and warmed up by the fireplace while I admired their different Christmas customs, with opening gifts in the morning.

Our Scouting leader, Paul Hokkeling was fatally injured on a Friday afternoon, about a year before Edward's dad moved the family back to the UK. I remember that day precisely, since our Scouting friend Piet was hit that *same* Friday, by a Dutch Army Jeep driven by drunk soldiers. His arm was caught in the side mirror, they hadn't slowed down. Edward and I both attended the Eindhoven Protestant Lyceum, but for one reason or another he had already left classes.

From the street across from the school, I witnessed Piet's accident. Our wonderful janitor and custodian, Mr. van den Waerden, saved Piet's life by applying a tourniquet. Piet kept hitting his ripped off arm with his hand, in shock and in disbelief. That Friday afternoon I called Edward that his friend Piet had lost his arm, and Paul was in a coma from lighting, while marching underneath Army barracks. The electricity landed on the metal roof, then on Paul. He never regained consciousness and died on Sunday.

Edward didn't believe me and hang up on me. Where were my parents, and why did it befall on me to make that most difficult of calls? By this time of course, Anita had been dead for a few years. Now it was Edward's time to make the hardest of phone calls: he cried and sobbed that Caroline didn't wake up that morning. We had all attended Paul's cremation, I'll never forget how Marjolein, his fiancé and Cub Scouting leader, had to be supported from grief when it came time to say goodbye.

* * *

A few weeks after Caroline's funeral I dried my tears, and left Holland. More than likely though, I had really wanted to leave home—and the fights with dad—behind. We'd been at war for too long. Stumbling upon academics as an adult was a gift; I fell in love with knowledge, despite, or maybe because of Aristotle. To prove him wrong, I worked hard for scholarships, trying to outstudy my physical challenges. I ended up doing weekly Paramedic shifts, taking patients to Detroit Receiving, William Beaumont Hospital and Pontiac, Michigan. It would take six days for my body to recover enough to do another shift; this was before automated Stryker frames. Some patients weighed 3-400 lbs., which was too much for my atrophied lower legs.

But since American flight medics had saved my life, I stubbornly yearned to pay back my cosmic debt. I'm still amazed that a high school dropout like me would graduate with honors from New Mexico Tech, especially since the skydiving accident resulted in a closed head injury. My willpower was both my strength and my weakness, and it brought me to my knees. Quite literally. Fast forward to that fateful year 2015, when I crawled through my home, incapable of walking a dozen feet. The devices that had served me after my discharge from the spinal cord rehabilitation hospital such as leg braces, cane, walker or wheelchair were no longer enough.

It felt as if I was walking on bones, which of course, was exactly what happened. In 1994, I'd even suggested a Rehabilitation Physician to inject silicone in my feet, to mimic the padding I had lost, but that wasn't medically feasible. After attending brilliant Physical Therapist/UNM Professor Dexter's lectures in 2006, the padding would be replaced by his painstakingly handcrafted, custom insoles. Other days, I could not stand upright as that brought on such severe lumbar back ache, I had to bend over within seconds.

It nags a little, to this day: had I pulled my reserve a second earlier, I would've been fine; a second later, though, and I wouldn't be writing this. Was it worth it, that I was rescued? That I survived? I don't know. But I am reminded of my accident every time my body cries its sad neuronal messages. *Your body is on fire! You're getting cut in half with a chainsaw! Right now, someone's hitting a sledgehammer on your sacrum!* All fucking day and night. It never ends, and the hardest part about it is that the skydiving accident, alone, did not cause this hell of an existence.

* * *

Without a doubt, the physical injuries I sustained after crash landing on Earth at 70 mph were extensive. The sacrum, at the bottom of my spine, was crushed, left more so than right, the last lumbar vertebra (L5) and the last thoracic vertebra (T12) were fractured, as were multiple ribs. I lost about two inches of my spine, L5 and S1 were shoved together. The cushioning between the two structures was removed when they fused, naturally—as opposed to surgical fusion.

The overall, initial damage from crushed and avulsed nerves directly lead to traumatic cauda equina syndrome, or CES.[40] This affects strength, sensation in the back of the legs and buttocks and hampers normal bowel, bladder and sexual function. 'Acute' CES is considered a dire medical emergency and may require immediate surgery. CES is especially difficult and devastating; although a patient appears able bodied, there is significant nerve damage that may even result in loss of anal sphincter tone, never a good sign. Realistically, a patient with CES may be able to walk behind a grocery cart that supports him/her for 10, 15 minutes but cannot stand in line for another five minutes, as collapse is imminent.

Some patients require catherization and bowel regime, much like patients with complete spinal cord injuries. The specific sensory deficits are described as *saddle anesthesia*, aka saddle numbness. The areas of your skin that are affected can easily be imagined by a rider sitting in a saddle. Someone with severe CES like me can be upright, yet my disability requires a soft chair, or lying down, within a minute.

Which is surprisingly hard to explain to a cashier or a store manager, never mind the general public, seeing someone walk from accessible parking to a motorized shopping scooter. Even with leg braces underneath my pants, or a cane, for over a decade I've always come across as *too* healthy, usually when I needed help the most.

Explaining all this is exhausting and hard to do, too, in the few seconds I had left before my body would give out. I've sometimes said to friends, acquaintances and even medical personnel that CES is like an *incomplete spinal cord injury*. Technically, that is not correct—the spinal cord ends at L1. However, what language is there to convey, and explain, the horse tail like nerve plexus underneath the spinal cord? People intuitively seem to grasp the concept of incomplete spinal cord injury, in situations where I did not have the energy or the patience to detail the difference between the spinal cord and the spinal cord roots. Never mind the concept of 'sacral nerve root avulsion.'

For my *severely comminuted* sacral fractures, surgery was never an option, with the crushed nerves. But of course, the tailbone never grew back right, either. It is now tilted at an angle, in a *sacrum acutum* position. Sitting has been painful since I broke my butt, and I suffer what I now know to be a 'sitting disability.' After living with worsening nerve and musculoskeletal torment for close to a decade—from 2005 to 2015—I was finally diagnosed with the progressive neuro-inflammatory disorder lumbosacral adhesive arachnoiditis.

Keep in mind that despite the textbook CES symptoms such as atrophied left calf muscle (the soleus, underneath the gastrocnemius) and bilateral foot muscles, the bladder, bowel and sexuality dysfunction, saddle numbness and severe sacral pain, it would take at least ten years post-accident before the diagnosis of cauda equina syndrome would appear in my medical charts.

* * *

To better explain adhesive arachnoiditis' *pathophysiology*—that's medicalese for 'the study of how shit hit the body's fan'—it helps to know a little about its anatomy. There are three layers of protective tissue around the brain, spinal cord, and the nerve roots, together they're called the meninges. The outer layer is the 'dura mater,' the middle layer the 'arachnoid,' containing blood vessels. The inner most layer is known as the 'pia mater,' Latin for 'small mother.' 'Dura mater' is akin to tough, or protective mother.

Adhesive arachnoiditis therefor is an inflammation of the fragile, middle layer, however it affects the dura layer as well. Two-thirds of the meninge are forever altered, with adhesions, or 'clumping' together of the nerves, the hallmark of this disease. The clumping causes scarring and inflammation, leading to further neurological alterations, such as Tarlov cysts, syringomyelia, tethered cord appearance, thecal sac abnormalities—a 2004 MRI clearly states *clumping and adhesions with probable arachnoiditis*.

The most significant consequence is dehumanizing pain that's treatment resistant and doesn't have a cure—although targeted treatment *may* alter its course, more research is needed.[41] The subarachnoid layer is tantamount; cerebrospinal fluid (CSF) circulates through and around the spinal cord and brain every two hours in the subarachnoid space. The CSF is responsible for providing nourishment to, and removing waste, from nervous system tissue. Adhesive arachnoiditis seems to cascade, and may contribute to other organ systems, e.g., skin, immune system and hormone, just like chronic regional pain syndrome, or CRPS. This is why personally, I prefer the term adhesive arachnoiditis syndrome.[42]

Conceivably, adhesive arachnoiditis can be provoked, or exacerbated, by multiple epidural steroidal injections—of which I had between 15 and 20 in an attempt to alleviate the CES pain. For all I know, it started with that fiasco of a lumbar puncture, or trauma from the sky diving accident. Other patients' adhesive arachnoiditis may have been triggered by a chemical, viral, bacterial or surgical insult to the arachnoid layer, or from an epidural during childbirth. However, as Dr. Tennant wisely reminds patients, "Don't waste time asking why, or how. You don't have the energy for it."

Progression of the disease triggers irreversible clumping that resembles overcooked spaghetti: the nerve roots below the spinal cord stick together, then suffocate. This specific damage not only worsens over time, the neuropathy—generated by the clumping, the scar tissue and inflammation of the nerve roots—also increases. Technically, this is known as 'lumbosacral adhesive arachnoiditis,' because it does not include the spinal cord itself (which terminates at L1-L2). You can see how it'd be much quicker and easier to explain one suffers from *spinal cord inflammation*, instead of saying *lumbosacral adhesive arachnoiditis.*

Every patient reports peculiar sensations, depending on the location of the inflammation, but most have in common severe lumbar backpain, leg pain and sensory alterations. Some patients have adhesive arachnoiditis of the cervical and thoracic spinal cord. An inability to stand is common for patients with adhesive arachnoiditis, it's therefor tantamount to investigate back pain with a neuropathic component. The inability to sit upright for more than twenty minutes is another clue. Personally, if I exceed my limits, it takes days, if not a week, to recover. I'm able to walk a very limited distance wearing my leg braces and using a cane, but after a few minutes, it feels like I'm walking on glass shards.

*   *   *

Recall that in 2005, Dr. Vos accurately diagnosed Brown-Sequard syndrome, which causes burning, electrical aches in the front and back of the left trunk, all the way to the pelvis. Although the hemangioma is located on the left side of the T4 chest level of the spinal cord vibratory sensation crosses to the right side of the lumbar and sacral plexus and thus, I have a diminished—or absent—vibratory sense on my right hip.

The longer I am upright, the worse the trunk pain—loss of spinal height means the ribs and hipbones are too close together rubbing one another, which aggravates the Brown-Sequard ache, and vice versa. I sure hoped the Brown-Sequard issue was the third, and hopefully my last, spinal cord lesion/injury! The torment resulting from the T4 hemangioma was diagnosed as 'central neuropathic pain syndrome,' or *central pain syndrome*.[43]

Central, because the damage originates in the central nervous system: the brain or spinal cord. Central pain syndrome can have multiple causes; for example, it will be experienced by twelve (!) out of every hundred patients with hypothalamic stroke. Central pain syndrome can be also be precipitated by epilepsy, multiple sclerosis, Parkinson's disease, tumors, sarcoidosis or spinal cord injury. Diabetic neuropathy, postherpetic neuralgia—persistent pain after shingles, phantom limb pain, trigeminal neuralgia and other diseases like CRPS may trigger relentless neuropathic pain and neuralgia.

Neuropathic pain is a huge, global problem: around 60-70 percent of diabetic patients and 20 percent of those with shingles will eventually present with neuropathy complaints.[44] Chemotherapy has also been known to induce neuropathy. Multiple studies found that 16-55 percent of back pain patients complain of a neuropathic component.[45] According to the must-read pocketbook *Neuropathic Pain*, this number is 25-30%. Many patients with back pain may not be receiving optimal treatment because their medical providers do not recognize the neuropathic component.

Neuropathic pain and neuropathy require a different approach than nociceptive pain such as arthritis, a fracture, soft tissue injury, or muscle cramps. Further, a lot of patients have mixed pain; both neuropathic and nociceptive. Interestingly enough, some researchers conclude that fibromyalgia itself may be precipitated by *small fiber neuropathy*. My impromptu hypothesis is that patients with irritable bowel syndrome—who interpret mild aches like bloating as severe, through no fault of their own—

maybe suffer from small fiber neuropathy as well.

I predict the next few decades are going to be disastrous: not enough patients with adhesive arachnoiditis, or even backache with neuropathy, will be identified in primary care settings. Adhesive arachnoiditis is seldom mentioned in medical school lectures, or any medical education. Current treatment modalities favor interventional therapies, such as back surgeries and epidural steroidal injections, which could lead to even more patients with adhesive arachnoiditis, or other neuropathy.

The peripheral nervous system includes all the nerves that exit the spinal cord, allowing us to feel and move our limbs. The central nervous system, as mentioned before, is composed of the brain and spinal cord. Neuropathic pain, whether *central* or *peripheral*, is excruciating. Think root canals, sciatica, or acute shingles. Typically, patients describe neuropathic pain as gnawing, burning, tingling, stabbing, radiating pain, or electrical sensations, and *the feeling of water dripping down their legs.*

Simply stated, in the brain, the thalamus and parietal areas are responsible for processing sensory stimuli. In a person with a normally functioning central nervous system, most do not notice—or find difficult—stimuli such as swimming in water, the breeze of a ceiling fan, showering, air conditioning or heat, the pressure of clothing on the skin, or sometimes, even one's own breathing. For someone with a central pain syndrome, phantom limb pain or CRPS, those sensations are interpreted as excruciating pain. The medical name for this condition is *allodynia.* [46]

* * *

Like many others who have—central—neuropathic pain, I experience the internal pain of the syndrome, but there's also the external sensory stimulants that agitate the nervous system. In my case, my skin feels as if I am dunked in a bath filled with ice cubes, but on the inside, it's as though someone pours molten lead, from T4 all the way down my spinal cord, to my toes. People with diagnoses and different histories might have different locations, or descriptions, of their pain. For anyone with a neuropathic pain component though, even the smallest movement or change in temperature can be excruciating.

Neuropathic pain causes another problem, *hyperalgesia*: a normally painful stimulus is perceived as extra painful. Between 15 to 50% of patients with neuropathic pain have both allodynia and hyperalgesia.[47] Sadly, neither

Complementary and Alternative Medicine nor Western, *allopathic* medicine provides significant enough relief for these types of neurological symptoms, also known as deafferentation pain.[48]

Neuropathy and neuralgia requires a trial of anti-seizure medications such as gabapentin (Neurontin), pregabalin (Lyrica) and/or the tricyclic antidepressant amitriptyline (Elavil). Side effects for these medications include drowsiness, dizziness, dry mouth and water retention, in almost ten percent of patients. Commonsense recommendations for medical providers and patients: start low, and go slow, and most importantly, *discuss realistic expectations*; gabapentin has an efficacy rate of around 30 percent, while pregabalin hovers between 35-50 percent.[49],[50] Individual differences are important to investigate; personalized medication, biomarkers and specialized pain medication therapy can ensure a much better outcome for patients. However, pharmacogenetic testing costs hundreds of dollars, isn't yet approved by the FDA, and for some medications genetic testing is not even available.

For patients it's hard to understand the inconsistencies within the FDA and government agencies. Epidural steroidal injections are a perfect example.[51] The FDA issued a 2014 warning about rare but devastating adverse effects of paralysis, death or stroke, while stating "that the effectiveness and safety of the corticosteroids for epidural use have not been established, and the FDA has not approved corticosteroids for such use."[52]

The FDA never approved steroids for injections into the epidural space, yet most pain clinics seem to use them, and since the 2016 CDC opioid guidelines, those injections are increasing. What sensible options do patients have? The providers who wanted to relieve my pain with epidural steroidal injections never disclosed the FDA's warning. The potential problems were made public, after patients started dying from an infected batch of methylprednisolone, used for epidural steroidal injections.

The first thing pain clinics and primary care providers—who haven't yet succumbed to the federal bullying and intimidation tactics—ought to do is an available saliva DNA test that may help determine a patient's rate of opioid metabolization. [53] Once provider and patient have this information, the patient can obtain appropriate and adequate analgesics, rather than becoming yet another victim in the out of control, politically driven *War on Opioids*.

Some patients are fast, or ultrafast metabolizers and may need much higher dosages of opioid pain medications. These genetic tests may not be failproof and not FDA approved, but right now there isn't an alternative: this beneficial test even shows your genetic response to over 40 other medications such as SSRI and tricyclic anti-depressant. The Millennium pharmacogenetic test is non-invasive and may avoid suicide, seen as the only way out by patients who are now forcibly tapered. If a lab test shows they are ultra-fast metabolizer, the battle is won.[54]

* * *

Most would think that the skydiving accident and my mobility aids were directly linked, but they were just the precipitating factors. In a way, my skydiving accident was never the worst of my problems. Perchance, I was. (Although various interventions, or lack of treatment, would tilt my fate towards adhesive arachnoiditis.) I pushed my body too much, often at the insistence of physical therapists and conventional wisdom in the pursuit of living a *normal* life. Having learned to ignore physical pain while mountaineering, I oscillated between taking it easy, which to me meant boring, and burnout from overdoing activities that were too strenuous.

But the damage from *not* treating the post-accident neuropathic and musculoskeletal pain surely contributed to my current central sensitization; a nervous system coming undone, firing painful message all the time.[55] After a month, I was medevaced from Riverside to Holland with a specialized bed by plane, in relatively stable condition, weighing my normal 118 lbs. While I was waiting for a spot to open up at a spinal cord clinic, I was admitted—condemned, really—to St. Ignacius Hospital.

The Dutch orthopedic physician was no Dr Cheng, and he heartlessly said, "Let's see how much pain you're in, we don't do morphine in Holland. Acetaminophen should be enough." I'm surprised he didn't hand out Louisa L. Hay's classic tome *You Can Heal Your Body*! Dr. Desmet kept his word and abruptly stopped IV morphine, without tapering. I almost died.

My American transfer sheet states: "Severe closed comminuted sacral fractures with distraction and marked angulation at the sacral vertebra #2; left ankle functional peroneal injury; perineal numbness—saddle distribution; no sphincter tone; post-traumatic stress; anemia secondary to blood loss with sacral hematoma; blunt chest trauma. L5 transverse fracture. Etc." I was transferred with an indwelling urinary catheter, because I was unable to void from the nerve damage.

The nursing team removed the catheter and shoved a metal bed pan under my—still fractured—buttocks and lower back. I cried when they closed the door and left me there, on the bedpan, then accused me of faking it. A day later, they finally inserted a catheter again. One month later I was transferred from St. Ignacius to the Lucas Clinic—according to Dr. Desmet's notes, in *good* condition.

I arrived at the specialized spinal cord rehab clinic in Hoensbroek, weighing 85 lbs., with hives from scalp to feet; traumatized, suffering severe, untreated PTSD, and I'd lost more than a pound a day. Dr. Desmet and the nursing team had neglected to provide Ensure, or extra protein, for the healing my body had to do—similar to burn victims—otherwise the body will literally eat itself, trying to make repairs. I would need catherization for six more months; the spinal cord clinic discovered another fracture, at T12.

* * *

Fast forward to two years *after* the accident: my limp, and the accompanying agony, had greatly worsened so I spend another six months at an outpatient rehabilitation clinic. The clinic had weekly, semi-mandatory sessions with a medical social worker. She had a kind face, and long, curly hair. After our third session she looked at me inquisitively and said: "I am really concerned. You are laughing inappropriately at serious, and deeply sad, family situations. Have you ever felt as if your boundaries were not intact, or affected you adversely?"

That's it, I thought. *I don't want to see this social worker ever again.*

Another time I was honest about what I experienced; I told a Physical Therapist there were shooting, sharp electrical pains, especially below the left knee.

"It feels as if my left foot is trapped in a meatgrinder, and the foot turns purple in the shower," I confided.

"That's great," she said, "That means the nerves are connecting again."

We continued the exercises, she urged me to *run* 20 meters, with my knees bent to ameliorate the fact I no longer had lower leg and foot muscles to push off on my toes. It's both a blessing and a curse to have an incomplete spinal cord injury. Because we are upright, we are told, by the medical establishment and well-meaning friends or strangers how lucky we are—compared to someone with a complete spinal cord injury such as paraplegia or tetraplegia.

Whenever patients with spinal cord problems over-exercise though, we risk harming the remaining neurons in the atrophied limbs, much like what happens with post-polio syndrome, or PPS.[56] I first made that link between incomplete spinal cord injuries and PPS in the early 2000s, after reading an article in *Scientific American*.

Did I take notice? Nope, just kept overdoing it, cheered on by misguided Physical Therapists. On a very practical level, just because I have an incomplete spinal cord, or spinal cord root injury doesn't mean I should carry heavy groceries and do home improvement projects, certainly not for decades.

* * *

A medical history is never straightforward, a patient's psyche and past medical, and life experiences, all contribute to the realm behind a clinical visit. At long last, after everything I have been through, it seems that this book was dreamt into existence; initially for myself, to understand my fate in this short life. But *The Queen of Ketamine* applies to everyone who feels like they've approached the end of their existence on Planet Earth. For everyone marginalized, pushed to the outer fringes of civilized society and excluded from enjoying a normal, productive life. Being alive with intractable, incurable torment—or another chronic disorder or disease—seems incompatible with *living a good life*. At least, the way it is defined by Aristotle, and my former Philosophy professor.

Because according to Aristotelian ethics, one needs 'good health in order to live a good life.' When I first encountered this philosophical idea years in Community College, I did not agree. Although, that was when I was in reasonably good health, limping along. If Aristotle is right, then why bother keeping this organism—myself—alive? For what purpose? With my health declining rapidly and the physical suffering increasing drastically, every annual document was titled "My Suicidal Year," and some *very* bad years were labeled "My Super Suicidal Year." I had struggled to hang in there, to keep my part-time job, to be a wonderful daughter, sibling, friend, student, girlfriend, and wife.

Behind the cheery façade and can-do attitude, it felt as though I was dying. Like many chronic pain sufferers, I'd reached the conclusion that this affliction had defeated me, utterly. The pain was always going to win. My particular torment may have been worsened by medical professionals who were supposed to help me, and yet, weeks before using the medications I'd hoarded for the purpose of ending it all, a handful of enlightened medical professionals tipped the balance and once again, saved my life.

One personal caveat: although a small dose of opioid medication—around 15-20 mg daily—helps with the deep, gnawing sacral pain, all too often, there are times when I end up moaning from anguish, immobilized with physical suffering. I've found that more opiate medications don't prevent this outcome, and sometimes, drugs just aren't enough to stop all the discomfort.

They help, but often cannot eliminate my affliction altogether. That's just the way it is. However, contrary to previous thinking and even the medical school lectures I attended, opioids *are* indicated for neuropathy and neuralgia. Research has shown that combining the anti-seizure medication carbamazepine and morphine may result in "less pain, and less opioids."[57] But the major painkiller, for me, would turn out to be ketamine.

5. ACCIDENTAL ANAL SEX & HUMAN COMFORT

As soon as I touched the mic I knew that's what I would do for the rest of my life. The big percentage is us, the real people, and we have to say something. You have to speak up. You have to. - Leslie Jones, comedian who makes fearless seem effortless

I didn't used to, but now I want, no demand, the same as able-bodied people. Happiness, friendship, community, love, sex. Cocks.

Well, the latter is a stage joke, but why not? Why can the *Sex in the City* characters yap about desire and male packages, but not *Sexy Crips in the City*? Come to think of it, where the heck *is* the dramedy *(c)rips in da City*?! Because I kid you not. I want it all, I want to live life.

When it comes to the disabled, however, society has yet to train us to see past the disability, wheelchairs and/or assistive devices to the human being right in front of you. Social media and activism have changed that a bit, but when is the last time you saw someone with a disability play a "normal" character in a Hollywood blockbuster who's getting it on? A story line that doesn't focus on disability or buys into the "super-crip" concept?

Buzzfeed contributor Laura Dorwart writes: "Stories often lean on disabilities as a way to propel narratives forward and provide conflict, rather than a concrete human reality."[58] Exactly. Compared to other minority groups, we have made zero inroads. It seems as if writer's rooms have no disabled staff members. Most characters with a disability are portrayed by an able-bodied actor, even for supporting and minor roles. Laura Dorwart writes "[…] only 2% of characters in the top 10 Nielsen-rated shows and the top 21 streaming original shows have disabilities. Of those characters, 95% are played by able-bodied actors."[59]

Or like we say: cripping it up! With 1 in 10 Americans suffering a severe disability, physically or mentally, this should be an outrage. "Speechless" was cancelled, "Breaking Bad" is over, and there isn't one TV drama featuring a cast member like Laura Innes' physician in *E.R.* using a crutch.

All we might remember is *House* and the portrayal of not just a "super-crip", but an addicted to opioids physician-super crip. That's the sad truth, and I've been a fan of Hugh Laurie since "Blackadder!"

We are the largest minority, so why aren't we represented on screen or in popular culture?

Years before Peter Dinklages' stardom, Jordan Prentice played a *midget on ketamine* (uttered by Colin Farrell's character) a gnarly American who snorted cocaine with Dutch hookers, in the brilliant black tragi-comedy *In Bruges.*[60] It's one of the best movies ever and *exactly* how a character with a disability ought to be portrayed. How did Martin McDonagh get it so right, and created Jimmy (Jordan Price), a layered, complex, real character?

So really, there is no excuse. Even without a disabled screenwriter, Hollywood limits itself.

Right now, can you name a female TV or movie character with disabilities, who has a normal storyline and how he or she deals with work, identity and sexuality? Mainstream media and magazines don't help, they rarely depict models with disabilities. One in five Americans have a disability—and one in ten a severe disability—yet their world, their reality doesn't exist. *My* world does not exist, except for Facebook groups, a few websites and the Rare Disease webpages of the National Institute of Health.

* * *

I had no female role models reflecting my disability, and had already felt quite disconnected for decades, remedied by running off into the mountains or pulling yet another geographical. My life hadn't been that happy, I dimly realized right after the accident happened. At that time, I'd roamed this planet for almost a quarter century, and I seemed to be perpetually on the run. During one of my most restless years I had lived in 10, 11 places, from the pre-gentrified Lower East Side, Williamsburg, Chelsea, Staten Island to Brooklyn Heights until I was back where I began, in Alphabet City.

Yet the more my body failed this Century, the better I understood the human need for comfort, for having someone by my side cheerleading. Having good relationships with family, friends, partners or lovers does give life meaning and purpose. I finally get it. Notwithstanding the fact that all of us are on a downward death spiral, our moments are fleeting and most likely we will die alone, the moments shared with other humans matter.

I may have had the insight that human connection is tantamount, yet I was quite lonely and as always, blamed myself. Despite performing comedy and working my butt off with new material, I didn't feel accepted in Albuquerque comedy yet. As though I was on the outside looking in, like I have done for most of my life. Perhaps a lifetime of bullying and choosing solitude had me so scarred, I was doomed to exist in a vacuum, on my own island, despite my gregarious nature and desire to be part of a community.

People tell me all the time how outgoing I am, but they don't know that most of my life is lived inside my hospital bed, and that I love being alone, too. I doubt that someone who is truly an extravert would be able to spend seven, eight or twelve hours a day alone, or do homework at New Mexico Tech's basement all day, without human interaction. I had to work hard, at Oakland Community College and Tech, since I wanted scholarships. Nevertheless, even then, I yearned to have friends, and a boyfriend. *And getting laid before I die.*

There were a few months, when I first started comedy, where it seemed the Albuquerque comedians welcomed me into their midst. For example, despite my physical discomfort and initial shyness at the mic during every performance at the Draft Station, I was invited to join a successful Monday open mic. I loved local comedy so much, I even threw an Annual Comedy Awards festival in March 2016, after collecting data via questionnaires all over town: Best Newcomer, Best Open Mic, Best Comedy Venue and Best Server. But not Best Comedian, that seemed like asking for trouble.

After a year of exhausting but exhilarating open mics and showcases, I would tell the "Fuck Oprah and her gratitude journals!" joke on stage at the National Hispanic Cultural Center, after accidentally heckling comic Natasha Leggero. Wrapped in my own bubble, oblivious to my surroundings, I'd yearned to send a quick text to another Albuquerque comedian, while Natasha was seconds into her set. My wheelchair and I were parked in the first row, and I freely admit that regardless of usually acting like an extravert, I do score a tad higher than most neurotypicals on the Autism Spectrum Disorder scale.

I was stoked sitting in front, next to Ann Gora's boyfriend. I always had trouble deciphering social cues. Or maybe, not understanding social nuances, had always provoked bullying. The preceding week I'd felt so lonesome, one year into my bedridden existence with less and less friends from my old life visiting. So, finally having a *comedian* friend to text was simply irresistible. Here was my big chance, and my baser instinct prevailed over common sense. Right after I pressed send, I got busted, badly.

* * *

"What are you texting?" Natasha Leggero asked, after sashaying over to face me directly.

"Eh, how wonderful Ann Gora's set was," I replied sincerely, as my only other comedy friend had opened for Natasha Leggero.

As usual, Ann had killed with her jokes on "checking out, via Xanax…the asshole thing to do though, it's gonna happen on a plane to Paris, while sitting in aisle seat. Have France deal with my corpse!" Her deadpan delivery and smart comedy are an irresistible combination.

"Yes, her set was great," Natasha replied.

I apologized profusely and put my phone away, then grabbed my notebook because was inspired to write a quip about Oprah. I also felt deeply embarrassed by the interaction and my behavior and had no way for dealing with it, aside from my notebook. My comedy notebook is my blankie, you see.

"Really? A notebook? What are you writing?"

"Eh . . . about Oprah," I answered truthfully.

"Well now, are you a journalist?"

"No."

"Don't tell me. Are you a comedian?"

Hesitant, "Nnn—Yes."

"Wanna come on stage and tell a joke?" she challenged me.

"Sure!" I replied, for once not hindered by my insecurities.

It felt like being back at New Mexico Tech, doing my own thing, and I hadn't realized that several comedians in the audience loudly yelled "noooo!" and "boo!" to Natasha. But she was the boss, so a buddy pushed me, in my wheelchair, up onto the stage. I halted, grabbed the spare mic, and was quiet for a second. Then I slowly turned on my purple LED wheelchair lights for both wheels, and began, "Now I'm ready!" to roaring laughter.

"So, I moved from Detroit to New Mexico, you know, for upward social mobility, to improve my life, yo. Moved straight from Detroit into a cute little home in a Socorro barrio, ese!" I quipped, then shared my favorite Oprah jokes, and was again rewarded with laughs. At the time, I had no idea who Natasha Leggero was, but she heckled me like a pro, and she was hilarious. After she and her husband Moshe Kasher's show ended, she said I did a great job. And that's how the first Oprah remark I'd scribbled after the spine doc told me to live *a very quiet and calm life with adhesive arachnoiditis* morphed into a future, comedic theme of holding Oprah responsible for the demise of humanity "and unleashing the four henchmen of the Apocalypse, Dr. Oz, Dr. Phil, Long Island fucking Medium, and of course, Deepak Chopra."

Later incarnations of the joke veered off into how Dr. Oz was destroying all credibility of gastroenterologist providers, with completely healthy patients worrying about their stool, "because Dr. Oz says it should be S-shaped" and how, if we ever met, "I would bitch slap the bullshit out of him." (Honesty dictates me to admit that although I came up with the four henchmen/Oprah joke, as an atheist it was an irresistible idea, but in a case of parallel thinking I later found the same idea online in a pro-science blog. I have an incredible memory, so it was most likely parallel thinking, because had I read it, I would have used a different analogy. Still, it doesn't sit right with me to not acknowledge that blog post, unfortunately I can no longer find it online but this post, on the dangers of fake medical claims is brilliant. [61]

The thing is, I wouldn't be so hard on Oprah if she sometimes had used her media empire for the advancement of science, or at the very least, occasionally had thrown in a 'vaccines are freaking awesome!' at one of her shows. Sadly, Oprah kept inviting anti-vaxxer dipshits like Jenny McCarthy. Anti-vaxxers base their belief system on a discredited and retracted Lancet Journal paper by Andrew Wakefield, who had lost his medical license, over said article! I'm not sure if she's an instrument of God or Satan, but she single-handedly convinced 60 million Americans, "To hell with your neocortex, feelings are everything." I mean, a seismic shift in the American ability to use logic happened, over the last twenty years.

Comedy kept making me happy: since my diagnosis, I hadn't stopped writing observations, monologues, and riffs to heal that internal abyss. I wanted to reach out, to whom or what I did not know yet, but I was contributing to a better life. Perhaps, Aristotle had not realized that comedy brings happiness, even to ailing bodies. Stanford has a nice overview of what Philosophy with a capital P had to say about humor: "Greek thinkers after Plato had similarly negative comments about laughter and humor. Though Aristotle considered wit a valuable part of conversation (Nicomachean Ethics 4, 8), he agreed with Plato that laughter expresses scorn."[62]

All my life, I'd tried so hard to belong, to befriend likeminded people, to connect to the world, to be productive and creative. Until I found comedy, I'd seemingly experienced nothing but failure, aside from my intermittent, intrinsic happiness within the provider-patient relationship. Most patients and I worked together so well, a true collaboration which contributed positively to their health and well-being. It was holistic, indeed: a good, old-fashioned common-sense attitude, paired with a dose of integrity.

A few months later, a professional Los Angeles comedian and actress would confide to me, "Natasha is hyper focused on not having her material recorded or written down, she—allegedly—once raged on an unsuspecting journalist, from the stage, who was there to do a profile" Having a smartphone, and then a notebook in my hand meant I was doomed, despite innocent intentions, generated by an overwhelming feelings of inadequacy and loneliness. Natasha had a good point though. Even in the Albuquerque community, some comics were known for joke stealing, especially from Twitter accounts.

With the comedy sets, a small sense of belonging, and a focus for my life, things were looking up. Besides, I persevered and accomplished the goals I'd set for myself in 2015. I got laughs, was offered a beer a couple of times, flirted like the end of the world was near, and even had a pump and dump. Go gimpy! I joked to my audience; "I'm a Type A gimpy. I don't know what else to do, can't imagine spending my life in a La-Z-Boy, watching Dr. Phil reruns and snorting oxycodone all day long." But it wasn't until my second year of doing stand-up that Nicole, one of my best, and oldest friends observed that comedy is what finally connected my heart to humanity, even more than being a Physician Assistant. Although, come to think of it, I did make patients laugh, a lot.

* * *

Back in 1993, when I was rehabbing at the Dutch spinal cord clinic, I became close friends with Rico Ramdhan and Raf Linmans. We teased each other mercilessly and made the lewdest and gimpiest jokes. When a few weeks later John Geven returned to the unit—the first time for his diving accident, this second time to recoup after his elbow tendon transfer surgery—he was told "One of the patients is a model." I wasn't well-known in Holland but had been on television and a few magazine covers.

Turns out John spent half the day looking for me with his manual wheelchair, which was slow going, with quadriplegia. Most patients were male, and two women over age 60, so it should have been really easy to find me. John actually had seen me, a few times. Finally, he had a PT session right across from me, nevertheless, it took his therapist to point at me, "That's her, she's the model you've been looking for!"

"Her?" John said incredulously, looking at my uncombed hair, my body clad in sneakers and baggy jogging pants. I had to show John a couple of magazine covers and pictures, because he still wouldn't believe me. I definitely was not a 'model' patient either, but at 24 years old my normal life had ended, so naturally I gravitated towards John, Rico and Raf, who were all a few years young than I. Boy, did we have fun. We even went to a nearby music festival where I had to fight with a group of drunk Swedes, who had stolen Raf's wheelchair. They wouldn't return the wheelchair, threw me their car keys and said I could have their Volvo.

Rico's neighbor Frans Meulbroek, an older, hilarious loudmouth truckdriver was our hero though. That dude was O.G. all the way. Our friend Michelle, from the upstairs amputation unit—who had lost her boyfriend and her legs in a car crash—climbed on Frank's face for oral sex, *every* night. We never knew if Frans, with C3/C4 quadriplegia would survive the night; his breathing was iffy even without Michelle sitting on his face! Afro-Dutch 17-year old Rico always gave me rides on his lap, when I was limping through the hallways with my cane, and it wasn't long before we started dating. My skydiving boyfriend had dumped me quickly after the accident and got back together with his ex, and I was extra susceptible to Rico's flirty demeanor and affection.

* * *

Alas, although I wanted sex, the damage had affected my sacral and lumbar plexus: the electrical impulses that should communicate between the lower half of my body and my brain no longer arrived, or if it did, the messages were fragmented. I have what a 'neurogenic bladder,' and do not feel my bladder expanding. Without feeling that urge to empty I have learned to pee every few hours. An average woman feels the need to urinate when she has around 250 cc in her bladder.

But my floppy bladder can hold over 1000 cc easily, and then overflow incontinence happens. Peeing ain't exactly normal either. I push urine out of my bladder via credating; placing a fist or stretched out hand into my lower abdomen/pelvic region. Dr. Crede was a European physician who first described impaired urination with a neurogenic, or 'floppy' bladder, and his namesake method is known as Crede maneuver. Sadly, that window into history seems to be lost forever, except for some old, digitalized spinal cord injury research papers.

I needed catheterization for the first seven to eight months post-accident, and I feel an intense gratitude for the ability to use a bathroom mostly independently. Bowels, same issues. Basically, my rectum and sigmoid colon are no longer receiving enough nerve signals for peristalsis, the natural movement which propels stool through the colon. Most people with complete spinal cord injuries catheterize and/or use MiraLAX or enemas to empty their bowels.

Others with a higher spinal cord injury like quadriplegia have incontinence and wear a condom catheter and bag or have a suprapubic catheter through the skin into the bladder. For my bowel care, I used digital stimulation if I haven't had a bowel movement in two days. I put on a glove and start digging —gently—or push from the outside, apply pressure to help pass the stool. Taking care of my abnormal bodily function can be quite tiring, as days turn to months and years, and the years inevitably into decades. It all takes so much time and energy.

* * *

At the time of my first rehab, I was confined to bed for three more months since another fracture was found, at T12 and from the severity of the sacral fractures. The Dutch spinal cord nurses had catheterized and evacuated my bowels for months. They got mad one day because the gang and I spent a fun night at the hospital basement bar, and we came back after curfew. Our favorite game was using Frans' face—immobile above his shoulders—as coaster throwing target, whoever hit him had to finish their beer at once. As punishment for coming in late though, the nurses refused to catheterize me until an hour and a half later.

They couldn't discipline my buddies in the same fashion, because they were either incontinent, or already knew how to cath themselves. I had terrible abdominal aches and was sweating while awaiting catherization. At midnight, after the next shift started, my bladder was finally emptied with an astounding 1450 cc. They were not happy, and they were displeased that I and my fellow patients were having fun, flings, and even sexual encounters.

A few months later, out of the blue, one day the nurses asked me to come to their station. "If only you'd behaved better, you'd leave two weeks later, but we want you out, now," head nurse Ratchett said with a satisfied smile, "start packing your stuff!"

To this day, not sure *why* I was kicked out prematurely. Was it because John, Raf, Rico and I had too much fun, playing chicken in the gym, going downhill at night falling out of our chairs, or perhaps, did I blab on Dutch TV how much I disliked the nursing staff, after how they treated me? Or was it because I'd smuggled in a little—legal—hash? *Oh, come on, I joke on stage, who doesn't smuggle in a little hash, being a spinal cord injury patient?!* Another one's of life's mysteries that will never be solved, I have long since lost the footage so don't even know what I said on the program. All I know is, I went back to the Spinal Cord Unit 10 years later with Jeremy when we were newlyweds at the tail end of our honeymoon, from Slovenia back to Holland.

I just wanted to be kind and say hello, as Jeremy and I would soon travel back to New Mexico. Well, let's say I left an impression, because some of them were *still* mad. After my almost year-long stint at the inpatient clinic, I finally went to adult education to obtain my high school degree. This cannot be equated to an American GED. The Dutch adult high school was an advanced placement equivalent, the last two years of high school condensed in one intense year, with mandatory all-day attendance. I biked back and forth from my accessible one bedroom, in the town I had left seven years earlier. I quickly found out that you can leave, but you can never come back.

By 1994 I found myself back in another rehabilitation setting, at an outpatient clinic. Around this time, I graduated Cum Laude from Eindhoven College, despite hanging out till the wee hours with my boyfriend, an Afro-Dutch DJ and rapper named Nathan de la Parra. I didn't take good care of myself those days, and did not realize that my witty, funny and talented black boyfriend was battling serious mental illness. Or that I was struggling myself.

* * *

Two decades later I am on stage myself, like Nathan once was, and I joke about spending the first half of the 2010s 'profoundly, deeply unfucked.' That's not the full truth, when I divorced in 2009 it would take seven years before I had sex again, in 2016. No sex for seven years? Dang, aren't I supposed to be at my sexual peak? The irony is not lost on me. I went on perhaps two, three dates after my divorce, and once in 2012, a British interventional cardiologist enthusiastically grabbed my breasts and shoved his tongue down my throat. I liked him, but there was no chemistry and he went too fast.

During those years, I didn't know that guys found my body attractive. Despite dozens and dozens of fashion magazine covers, and that ill-fated modeling career in my teens and twenties, I had never felt at home in my old modeling and stunt woman's body, and now lived in a new body I disliked even more. I didn't have low self-esteem, I had no self-esteem at all when it came to dating. The only features I liked about myself were my nose and my legs, and we all know what happened to my legs. Which left my nose.

Seriously, my all-natural nose is beautiful, and outfitted with an above average sense of smell. My nose is so drop dead gorgeous, Nicole Kidman wished she had my nose! Of course, the best nose in Hollywood is Angela Bassett's, wished I had hers, but that would look weird. Look, my point is that you can't buy a nose like mine, not even from the best plastic surgeon. And it's virginal! It's never snorted cocaine, ecstasy or ketamine, for example. My cartilage is outstanding.

Aside from liking my nose though, I exuded zero sexiness. I'd perfected a boyish, don't-even-look-at-me attitude, which, combined with having very little confidence, no doubt negatively affected my modeling and stunt career. I could not sell sex. One needs to feel sexy on the inside to exude sexy on the outside, and this applied to dating too. Since the accident, I had only slept with Nathan, and Jeremy.

Convinced I wasn't good in bed, I took love and sex out of the equation and focused on work, home improvement projects and an Ikea-kitchen. I felt ambivalent about sex, too many guys had leered at me since childhood. I was preyed upon, and of course, there was date rape, a girl's rite into womanhood, at age 16. Which is in one of my sets, and it's funny, since you know, I'm taking back the power.

"Amazing insights happen after you survive a serious accident. There I was, dying in the desert, and when I came to, the first thing that came to mind was: Whoa….date rape….definitely not the worst thing that has ever happened to me! Anyway, I was in the middle of getting date raped, and this douchebag goes, 'would you like to have sex with two guys?' 'Nah, thanks, I'm good, I'm kinda busy and usually one dude suffices.' Look, guys, don't judge me, you haven't partied on Ibiza unless you've been date raped by a tall Spaniard who looked like Fabio. The worst thing was, he was too cheap to roofie me and now I have to remember his weird, red little bratwurst, for the rest of my life!"

One of my best buds, Francisco, laughs so hard at this joke, complete strangers, women, get mad and asked their boyfriends to beat him up, because apparently, one oughtn't make fun of date rape. Ironically, in Milan my Canadian friend Martina had a nasty situation, allegedly, with the real Fabio. What?! Truth, right? Always beats fiction.

* * *

Before I perform that joke, I even say, *trigger warning*. Weirdly, I can do the date rape joke no problem, yet I hadn't yet been able to joke about the day a big, muscular boy of 14 covered my 11-year-old body with his, at a near-deserted beach. I had yelled 'help' to my younger sister and brother who were playing next to us in the sand, but they ignored me while the boy demanded *a real kiss*. Eeeew. Keeping me pinned down for what seemed like hours, he opened his mouth, saliva dripping slowly to my lips, which wasn't the worst: regretfully I ended up carrying this shameful feeling in my chest.

Days later I finally told my mom, rambling that he was on top of me, so it was as if *we were having sex* and he'd force me to kiss him, and she said: "Oh honey, don't feel bad." The salty seaside air was howling when we walked next to each other, in our rubber boots, carrying shovels—sadly *not* for burying his dead body. Did she hear me? Perhaps our words had drifted off by the Autumn winds, all the way across the Atlantic to where the Six Million Dollar Men lived. Decades later she apologized for not beating up the little shit, who wrote me letters for months. Heartfelt apologies are part of a Hero's Journey, and I gladly accepted my mom's. In 2006, in tears, I would apologize to my little sister for abandoning her when I moved to Paris.

One thing I knew for sure: I had been loved, truly loved at least once, this lifetime. So, occasionally I got on match.com or Tinder yet was sure I would leave this life profoundly, and deeply underfucked. That's so sad. Not surprisingly, I had no luck whatsoever with dating apps. Without confidence, but now much more disabled, my dating and sex life became a self-fulfilling prophecy. Although things were looking up when I finally had another hilarious, meaningless one-nighter. Go gimpy! Nevertheless, I thought I'd never have a long-term sexual relationship again.

Isn't it remarkable how our societal myths also get in the way of knowing the reality behind all the labels and boxes? Not just for folks with disabilities, who want to have sex too. For instance, did you know that most male, gay couples—over 60 percent—don't do anal? [63] There's lots of mutual masturbation, genital stimulation, oral sex, and kissing though. Get this: half of straight males and females are having anal sex.[64] But gays were banned from donating blood for decades, primarily for the perception of anal sex and HIV transmission.

That's why New Year's Eve 2016 was the stuff of legends, about two months in the making. In September that year, I had checked out Craigslist to see if there was a good match, at first in the casual encounters section, cuz I was pretty happy with a toot it & boot it. But that was the most gruesome sausage fest, so I quickly went for the men seeking women section. This nice guy posted he'd like "to have a cup of coffee and take it from there." Oh, yes, I wanted to take it from there!

I couldn't tell where Dylan was from, didn't care, but he had brown skin and the most beautiful, dark, slightly slanted eyes. I felt a flutter, as he seemed really sweet. We met on Saturday, October 29 at Deep Space Coffee, and it was lovely. We kept seeing each other twice a week and had sex on our fifth date. It was as if we went on a hot date once and then those wonderful, amazing dates just kept hot happening. Dylan Tsosie and I had a lot in common, as struggling artists working on our first large scale, serious projects.

I'd already started my memoir, and Dylan painted contemporary life on the Rez, a series of eight oil paintings in a style called Western Realism. "I don't like that cliché, on the nose thing, with Natives on horses, with feathers, fighting in some battle. I paint horses in the landscape, or my family and our get togethers through old photographs," Dylan said on our first date. Dylan's fascination for European classical painters, and his Fine Arts education is evident from the way light radiates from his subjects and the landscape.

One of my favorite paintings is "Cook-Out," one person is shooting, another lights a fire, there's a forlorn metal chair, all set against the phenomenal nature of the Navajo lands. That painting reminded me of my family's make do attitude. Where I am from no one eats roadkill. Ever. But we did, after killing an old, large rabbit on a small road near the ocean behind the dunes, and we ate fish from mountain streams. My siblings and I also literally scavenged, we'd attack and inhale leftovers from diners before us, if a mountain hut served hot food.

*　*　*

On December 31st, I decided we should celebrate New Year's in fashion. I got some LED candle lights and queued up a Netflix comedy to watch from my twin sized hospital bed. My house by the way has no fucking Feng Shui. Literally. There is no transition from making out to doing the sweet stuff. I have two gorgeous club chairs and the hospital bed, but there is no kissing on the couch before sex, as I didn't have a couch.

For the first time in my life though, I felt so sexy; I even went to Wal-Mart to buy lacy underwear. It turns out that Wal-Mart shoppers want to be sexy too, but not at Victoria's Secret prices. The labeling on their undies are hilarious, and I bought three skimpy lace panties labeled My Secret Garden. *I don't think it was a secret for long though, that my garden was getting plowed!* I also joked to the audience: "A comic once asked me, does everything work below the waist? Yes! Works-below-the-waist is my Tinder handle. I'm just kidding, my Tinder handle is Sex-On-Wheels!"

After Dylan and I had sex for the second time that evening, on that New Year's Eve I'll never forget, the weirdest pillow talk, ever, ensued.

"Dylan, did we just have accidental anal sex?"

"Wouldn't it have been harder to push it in?"

"God, is there a millennial who hasn't had anal sex?"

"Eh . . . it wasn't that good anyway."

"Oh. My sphincter is kinda kaput, so we wouldn't have noticed."

It was an easy mistake to happen. It was dark, I have little to no feeling of the superficial skin receptors. Also, we were spooning, because that's how all crippled people have sex. Just kidding! I was tired and on steroids from the spinal cord inflammation flare up. Despite the fact I am not that adventurous in bed, I was stoked. I felt victorious; two one-night stands earlier that year, and then, one long hot relationship going, and to top it off, I may have had accidental anal sex on New Year's Eve. Who knew I'd finally get to a place where sex was not only possible, but enjoyable, too?

I did make Dylan promise to be the guardian of my holes from that point forward. I liked this guy, although it's hard to find a couple that differs more, in character and personality. I'm extremely outgoing and appear confident, despite deep-rooted insecurities, and he is super introverted, shy and yet, secure in his ability as a great oil painter. Man, I dig this dude so badly. Dylan usually tries to get away with as few words as possible, so the night ended like this:

"Dylan, let's never speak of accidental anal sex ever again."

"OK."

"Except when I do stand-up three times a week!"

"OK."

6 ROMAN POLANSKI, DMT & A LOT OF HIPPIES

My life seemed to be a series of events and accidents. Yet when I look back, I see a pattern. - Benoit Mandelbrot, mathematician & fractal celebrity

Oh Albuquerque," I quip in my stand-up routine, "I hate your weed!" Seriously, I loathe an altered state of consciousness so much, I don't partake in weed, or do edibles. And not just because New Mexico stoners can't keep their story straight on the shit they're smoking. As soon as I had rolled up in my manual wheelchair and waded through a platoon of funky looking hipsters and ill-smelling hippies, at least four glass pipes were offered to me. I smiled and said "No, that stuff worsens my pain! Thanks though."

"You're gonna do fine, it may help if you smoke sativa. Or indica?" said Nate, looking mightily confused, "Hey Joey, was it indica or sativa that does the body high and keeps your mind happy?" They meant well and were sweet, the kind of hippies I did tolerate. But I wasn't even tempted to try a whiff of that ill Burque shit. They'd all gathered for an epic djembe drumming circle in a friends' backyard, to celebrate a full moon. It was one of the last times I would go to a private residence, with my minivan and manual wheelchair. I'd tried medical weed once or twice since the torment got bad, but it always worsened the neuropathy.

Hardcore stoners wore me out too, after a while they all sounded the same. Besides, I can't play djembe—although I did have so much fun trying. I'm not against weed, or hippies, though. In my Libertarian opinion, weed should be sold at Walgreens. Let's finally cut out the baby killing cartels!

Because I was very Libertarian about illicit substances in my sets when I first started comedy, the audience offered me drugs afterwards. In my stand-up I quip that "My main post-apocalyptic survival skills are great blowjobs, and suturing skills, but it doesn't hurt to have a stash." And no, there's none left, being gregarious I gave away all of the acid and mushrooms. away.

Seriously though, my main justification for partaking in recreational drugs, aside from wanting to stay sober were the vicious drug cartels. From a young age, I was aware of the brutal and murderous criminal organizations. I was the kind of kid in the neighborhood collecting 25 cents for baby seal rehabilitation centers, when their kin were getting clubbed for their fur. As a Dutch teen, I figured that if no one in the US used illegal drugs, more men, women, and children would remain alive, South of the border.

Perhaps naïve, but for me the only logical, ethical and humanistic stance until homegrown weed and American-made psychedelics and recreational drugs will finally disrupt the cartels' monopoly. Decades later, despite the rise of US laboratories and *organically* grown weed, sadly the cartels aren't killing fewer people. PBS' *Frontline* states that "between 2007 and 2014 there were 164,000 homicide victims in Mexico," compared to 103,000 civilian deaths in Afghanistan and Iraq during the same time period.[65]

* * *

Within days of moving to Paris, Gerald Marie, the infamous Elite Plus Models owner/booker, had offered me a joint—the European name for a tobacco cigarette with weed or hash. I'd asked for a glass of milk instead, because I'd quit smoking hash a couple of months ago, after Caroline had died. Everyone made fun of me; Gerald, still married to supermodel Linda Evangelista, laughed the hardest. At seventeen, despite feeling lost in my life, and my own self, I felt mightily out of place among these jokers.

Suffice it to say I wasn't known for partying, as I usually disappeared into the mountains when I wasn't working. Oh how I longed for those days, carrying a 34-pound backpack with a tent, sleeping bag, food, water, and a First Aid kit during strenuous, but beautiful solo hikes in the French Alps. I would later switch to Karin Models and met notorious owner Jean-Luc Brunel a couple of times. Modeling agency owners, bookers and their rich friends were all the same. Uber-douchebags trying to bribe young, underage girls, just like—allegedly—Prince Albert of Monaco, with whom I once shared a cab from a fashion show to the Bain-Douches nightclub.

Later that night, his sister Princess Stephanie danced on a table in front of me, making weird, lewd jokes. One evening I saw Roman Polanski at Les Bains, seemingly with Francis Ford Coppola. A young girl was sitting on Polanski's lap, we can only hope that was his future wife, Emmanuelle Seigner. Maybe Roman and Francis weren't close friends, but merely circling in the same orbits: Roman's *Chinatown* lost an Oscar to Francis' *The*

Godfather II. They had been part of the same up and coming filmmakers in sixties' Hollywood.

Francis Ford Coppola's reputation, however, is impeccable. His oldest son, the talented Roman Coppola was born in France in 1965. Roman has skirted around the name-issue but admitted his dad looked up to Polanski in a 2002 interview.[66] Reality, right? Always weirder than fiction. In 1977 Polanski had been charged with six felony counts in Los Angeles, five counts were dropped in exchange for a plea bargain. The deal he cut left the *least* serious of all charges, sex with a minor aka statutory rape—including oral, vaginal and anal penetration with the 13-year-old. A then 43-year-old Polanski fled rather than awaiting sentencing, since France doesn't have an extradition treaty.

Come to think of it, that's why France was also the perfect country for sex crimes against American minors, those underage, young models, or as Polanski describes teenage girls: nubile. Since Polanski had pled guilty to all six felony counts, the statute of limitations doesn't apply, but it's much more complicated than space will allow me here. I refer you to Jeffrey Toobin's excellent article "The Celebrity Defense." [67] All six charges, including 'rape by use of drugs' and 'furnishing a drug (Quaalude-KG) to a minor' are therefore pending, and an arrest warrant waiting.

Whoopi Goldberg said in 2009 that Polanski was not guilty of *rape-rape* and Hollywood stars Woody Allen, Tilda Swinton, Martin Scorcese and a hundred others signed a petition on behalf of their famous friend, when he was detained in Switzerland. Good Lord, what was their defense, Polanski's movie *The Pianist* was so great?! Quentin Tarantino famously denied it was rape: "She wanted to have it and dated the guy. The girl was down with this." Harvey Weinstein adamantly defended his friend, and Hollywood stars from Kate Winslet to Jodie Foster and Harrison Ford performed in Polanski films. Polanski was even given a cameo in Rush Hour 3, starring Chris Tucker and Jackie Chan.

"Hollywood has the best moral compass, because it has compassion," Harvey Weinstein once told the Los Angeles Times—the article was taken off-line by the LA Times, but there are multiple references to it.[68] The Weinstein Company produced *Roman: Wanted and Desired*. It's an exculpatory documentary if you think he should do at least a month at San Quentin and profess a public apology, or not exculpatory enough, if you believe the American justice system was out to get Roman.

In 2009, the Huffington Post published an eerily clairvoyant essay, "Wonder Why Middle America Doesn't Trust Hollywood Liberals? Three Words: Weinstein and Polanski." [69]

* * *

Interestingly, and not even known online, is the fact French modeling bookers, playboys and agency owners such as Jean-Luc Brunel—one of Jeffrey Epstein's friends—wouldn't have been very successful in sweet-talking teenagers on their own. They were ugly, old assholes, even way back when in the eighties. Those guys were smart, they had their early-twenties, handsome but impoverished buddies groom and love bomb the girls they wanted, for themselves or for their friends.

I nicknamed those guys *dogs* and some of them were actually okay, especially since I didn't play the game. The fact is, they send the dogs in first, to establish the con. Because all this abuse, from the casting couch to using date rape drugs, everything those hucksters do is a con. Weinstein et all are conmen. They get off on using, abusing and breaking young females, with quintessential conman tactics. The girls are marks, targets. One of the young dogs—allegedly—was super-duper handsome Jean-Yves Le Fur, a *real estate broker* and Princess Stephanie of Monaco's fiancé in 1990.[70] I personally never saw Jean-Yves work in real estate, he seemed busy brokering and procuring girls for his rich and influential patrons. Allegedly.

I recall listening in on a conversation by two older dudes, that Jean-Yves himself was instructed to use Stephanie for her Monaco real estate connections—again, allegedly. I was always listening, no one suspected the charming girl with blond braids who drank milk kept records. In 1993 Jean-Yves became Karen Mulder's fiancé—she was a Dutch top model who had a very public nervous breakdown and was involuntarily committed. Her psychiatric stay was paid for by Gerald Marie, whom she'd accused in many interviews as raping her. Gerald Marie himself was later caught bragging about banging 15-year-old teens in modeling contests and offered 300 pounds for sex with a minor, in a BBC undercover documentary. Nice lad, that.

In the summer of 1986, Karen and I shared the same apartment building around the corner from Avenue de L'Opera, near Elite Plus. The fancy building housed female models and we paid the agency back every month. The fancy studio complex was owned and managed by Frenchmen Michel, who drove a *Maserati*—I'm a minivan expert, couldn't care less about fancy cars but my Dutch friend Frank loved that car. Michel and Karina, his 1.80-meter-tall model girlfriend were so nice, I really liked them. While they went out partying, Frank and climbed out of the attic on to the Parisian rooftops, conquering entire city blocks.

Refusing that first Parisian spliff and asking for a glass of milk was a smart move: in ten years of modeling not only was I never offered cocaine, I wasn't offered *any* drugs by industry insiders. In stand-up I quip, "You know how unpopular I was, as a model? I was never offered coke, ever!" My clean-living reputation protected me, but of course, may have hindered a more lucrative career. Whatever. With hindsight, the old guys probably didn't like me joking in their face about them still going to Les Bains in their wheelchairs, with a care attendant, in another decade.

Yet I had been overdosing on a particularly addictive, and perhaps, much deadlier drug than cocaine: adrenaline. Before my accident, my life only seemed worth living if death was a split second away. In my case, it might have been safer to snort the occasional cocaine, then jumping out of planes. Being in front of an audience doing a good set and making people laugh was much like an adrenaline rush, but a happy one. It's a total endorphin high, comparable to reaching the top of a mountain after an arduous three-day solo climb. Except of course, without the risk of dying, even if I bombed.

* * *

Despite comedy and moving downtown to be nearer to a heated pool—the water in public pools had become too cold for me—I once again wished Bad Spot Bill hadn't phoned the trauma helicopter. Was it a blessing or a curse that I was alive after that horrifying accident? Because after twenty plus years of smarting, each year brought more agony than the one before. Grief, over the loss of my legs, career, marriage, and freedom was never complete. As you now know, adhesive arachnoiditis pain has rightfully been compared to that of having metastatic cancer, but without the relief of death; this amount of suffering, without an expiration date, seems unjust.

Life was moving me faster and further away from the accident, but I seemed fated to become a full-time patient, and not part time, as I'd like it to be. It wasn't just the spinal cord rehabilitation in 1992/1993, I had also rehabbed in 1994 when my gait worsened, and pain levels soared. Even at my beloved New Mexico Tech I had to skip a semester or two, from physical burnout—not that I would ever have an inkling into my wellbeing. I was so clueless, had quite possibly zero insight into my own health.

After my graduation in 2003 I was honored to be accepted at Quinnipiac, one of the best PA schools in the country with a fantastic director, Cynthia Booth-Lord. Like usual, I didn't have the right tools in place for my disability, physically or mentally. In a fit of optimism, feeling as if my body had improved a little, I donated my super lightweight, Dutch manual wheelchair to Jeremy's friend John. John's cousin had been without health insurance, the girl was 19 and after an accident was using one of those American clunkers.

"Are you sure?" Jeremy asked me, concerned. "Oh yes, I'll be just fine!" I replied, in total denial. I was probably trying to simplify my life, as my 2-bedroom mobile home didn't have a storage shed. The grueling move to the Connecticut PA school, when I hadn't yet recovered from the physical demands of the Tech Bachelors, meant I had to withdraw after the summer semester. The classroom was upstairs, my bookbag was heavy, and I no longer had that spiffy lightweight wheelchair. Quinnipiac was keen to keep their beloved, valued student and offered me a spot again in 2004. I was beyond exhausted, all the time, and although I could not see it then, I had been worn out since the skydiving accident.

By the time 2004 came around, instead of almost starting my second year at Quinnipiac, I had attended Gaylord's out-patient rehabilitation three times a week. When Jeremy was offered a job in Bernalillo after finishing his Master's, we decided to move back to New Mexico. Connecticut also seemed a little backward, in bookstores Native Americans were classified as Indians, and in general, Connecticut appeared a tad snooty. We had been happily living in our black, impoverished Hamden neighborhood, and had friends among our neighbors and landlady, yet couldn't wait to get back to *civilization*.

* * *

It seemed that every decade, heck, every year, I had to say goodbye to more and more *normal* body functioning. Since the summer of 2016, a new, different sensation had manifested. It felt as if a buzzing, electrified soundwave pierced my body, as if I was leaning against one of those Dutch farmer's electrical fences with non-lethal shocks, that keep the cows corralled. This was a symptom I absolutely could not live with.

Most likely, the adhesive arachnoiditis had worsened, or flared. Perhaps the adhesions themselves had worsened. That made sense, as the back of my legs now often felt as if there was water trickling down, a common complaint of adhesive arachnoiditis and neuropathic pain patients. I assumed it was a bad, but not irreversible, flare-up, and my friend Forrest Evans took me to an Urgent Care after posting a FB message, or rather, a cry for help.

"We can't give you pain medications, you know?" said the Google Glass wearing NP when she entered the exam room.

"I know, don't want or need any, but I would really, really like a short course of steroids," I replied softly.

I received methylprednisolone, a steroidal medication for five days, which helped a little.[71] Yet, I yearned for solutions beyond, or in addition to my current medication regimen. My neuropathy and neuralgia weren't even well controlled on the following regimen, immediately after a 12-day rehabilitation hospitalization in 2015:

- Oxycontin ER—extended-release—10 mg twice a day, a DEA Schedule II medication. This

  long acting opiate did seem very effective for the severe, deep arthritic pain of the old sacral, vertebral, and rib fractures.

- Oxycodone/acetaminophen IR—immediate-release—5mg/325 mg, half a tablet once or twice a day, aka Percocet, for breakthrough pain, also Schedule II. Oxycontin, the long acting version worked so well, I hardly ever needed more than five to ten mg daily of the IR medication.
- Gabapentin 800 mg four times a day. Gabapentin is an old antiseizure medication with a comparatively high safety profile, I've taken it for over 15 years without side-effects—although I have to watch my weight and keep swimming.
- Baclofen 20 mg five times a day; a common spinal cord injury medication for muscle spasms.
- Aspirin 325 mg four times a day. I like aspirin better than acetaminophen (Tylenol) or ibuprofen (Advil, Motrin). Generic aspirin is cheaper and doesn't upset my stomach or esophagus.
- Xanax—alprazolam—0.125 mg, a Schedule IV medication. Occasionally, once a week at most, if baclofen does not alleviate

spasms enough, I break a 0.25 mg tablet in half.
- Amitryptiline 75 mg at bedtime; to help with sleep, neuropathic pain and depression.

Regarding opioid medications, I thought—naively perhaps—there hardly would have been an opioid *epidemic* had medical providers been instructed by their medical boards to prescribe an immediate-release opioid with this simple warning: "Only use your IR opioids when you truly have breakthrough pain, when it's a 7-8 or higher, or it will no longer be as effective. Also, here is a DNA mouth swab test to see if you are a fast, poor or normal metabolizer." For years I strongly suspected I was a 'poor' metabolizer, as I seem to get by with a relatively low dose.

There doesn't seem to be an opioid epidemic—at least not the kind shoved down our throats by the media—there are contributing factors. What we certainly got is an epidemic of people taking opioids with multiple medications, adding alcohol and other, illegal drugs on top. What we do have is an alcohol epidemic, that is starting to effect millennials. I blame those hipster beers with ridiculously high alcohol percentages. Millennials are now dying of liver cirrhosis in record-breaking numbers. Every movie or TV show has female characters downing copious, ludicrous amounts of wine in huge glasses, as if that ought to be the norm.

Where *is* the outrage over the *nicotine epidemic*, which kills almost half a million Americans a year, where is the joint effort by media to address alcohol deaths, at 88,000 annually? Besides, most of the so-called opioid deaths are by people who did not take their medication as prescribed. Seriously, because who cooks their Fentanyl patch and injects it? Not chronic pain patients. And how many of those opioid deaths are suicides, ironically by patients whose pain clinic closed, or whose primary care provider office has been bullied by the government *guidelines* and consequently no longer prescribes opioids?

The Law of Unintended Consequences never fails. Patients who were on a stable regimen are denied access and may turn to heroin or illegally obtained opiates. That is not an opioid crisis, but another iatrogenic consequence. Why, instead of rushing those CDC Guidelines through, was the extent of the *crisis* not researched? Why not encourage providers to give every patient that Millennium pharmacogenetic test, to see if a patient is a fast or slow metabolizer? Very few deaths are caused by opioids only, most are *mixed drug use* deaths. New York City features meticulous Medical Examiner officers who properly record what people die from: over 90 percent from multiple drugs, mainly illegal fentanyl, benzodiazepines and alcohol.[72] Patients with chronic pain, using their opioid prescription exactly as instructed are *not* the problem.

To complicate matters, in Europe, the lowest available dose of Oxycontin —the long acting opioid—is 5 mg, instead of 10 mg. This worked well for me, until the spinal cord inflammation finally tipped me over a threshold into agony 24/7. But why is it that the brand name Oxycontin can be prescribed at 5 mg in Europe, while America's lowest prescription dose is 10 mg? All I needed was 5 mg, twice a day to control for the residual pain in the lumbosacral area. After the 12-day hospitalization in November/December 2015 at Lovelace Rehabilitation, I was told to take 10 mg twice a day. That's on you, America!

Sometimes when I see things I don't like, I point my finger at America and ruminate; *America, this America right now, not the gung-ho, hardworking, and optimistic America of twenty years ago, seems to have morphed into a nation of wusses. I wasn't even prescribed any opioids after I broke my leg in 1991! And of course, I did not want to take Oxycontin at twice the dosage I had used safely before. What am I, an American? Mmm . . . I must admit the long-acting medication does help with the deep, gnawing sacral anguish, as I hardly need any instant relief opioid medication for breakthrough pain. I'm also able to sleep through the night. Maybe being an American isn't so bad, after all.*

* * *

Another issue I seriously grappled with was insurance. My BCBS Medicaid plan refused to pay the long acting pain medication which was at least $400 a month. Unfortunately, the fucking dipshits from Walgreens failed to tell me that after it was finally approved via Prior Authorization, I ought to submit paperwork for the three months I paid the medications myself and it would have been reimbursed. When they finally told me eight months later, I couldn't submit a claim any longer. There goes another $1200, when being disabled is already expensive!

There is nowhere to go with my anger about the incompetency I've encountered as a patient. Whether it was the American or British medical providers who probably should never have injected epidural steroids near already scarred lumbosacral nerves, or the Pharmacy techs and home health care givers, or the ER physician who injured me with a botched lumbar puncture. I recalled how my body screamed *Noooo Kaatje!* before she started the procedure. The pain during that lumbar puncture was almost worse than the skydiving accident, my left leg immediately felt as if it was on fire.

I do blame myself for not listening to my intuition, especially since I worked at Socorro General as a Nursing Tech. I knew this doc. The kind of person who takes an entire pizza from the staff room, without ever bringing food or a treat themselves. It was undeniable. The sheer parade of greedy, uncaring twats I've met in my 20+ year journey through health care makes my mind and body feel as if I'm on a perpetual Disneyland Space Mountain ride. One that does not end well, with carts careening out of control. But I blame myself most, for not listening to my gut. It seemed I never learned from my mistakes.

No matter what, I seriously would have been better off without invasive medical treatments, had I found right medical marijuana, or perhaps micro-dosed psychedelics instead—a small dose that does not get you *high* or causes *hallucinations*. Already, much-needed research at Imperial College and University College London shows promise by using MDMA aka 'ecstasy' for depression, PTSD, and alcohol use disorder. Micro-dosing psychedelics may even help with end of life issues, as it can help put your life in perspective.[73] Wouldn't it be nice to feel at peace—instead of bitter, frightened, and remorseful—during your last seconds on Earth?

Sometime in 2017 I'd met a New Mexican teacher who confessed to micro-dosing mushrooms three to four times a year, to control her cluster, aka *suicide* headache. A nice, decent human being who unfortunately would get fined, jailed, and certainly lose her job had the State known about this. Psilocybin—magic mushroom—is another Controlled Substance, Schedule I even, on par with heroin and LSD. You gotta take everything the US government does with a grain of salt: psilocybin and LSD are classified as *highly addictive and serve no medical purpose.*

* * *

The Multidisciplinary Association for Psychedelic Studies (MAPS) deserves a Congressional medal, for their decades of persistence.[74] Thanks to them, the FDA approved a MAPS' Phase II clinical trial to evaluate MDMA-assisted psychotherapy for Post-Traumatic Stress Disorder, or

PTSD. Even Stars and Stripes magazine applauded their research and emphasized the great socioeconomic burden of PTSD in veterans.[75] Sporadically, the VA uses IV ketamine but only after first, second and third lines of treatment have failed, or suicide is imminent—veterans have a suicide rate of 22 a day.[76]

Despite my Libertarian pro-drug stance, I had yet to trip balls, and I was too scared to take the MDMA offered to me at High Mountain Hideout, a festival near Taos in 2015. The good old days, when I deludedly thought myself camping was still possible, as long as I slept in my minivan. That weekend was a nightmare. I was in so much pain, despite leg braces, orthopedic boots, canes, and my wheelchair. It was cold and the terrain not suitable.

An inebriated hippie with a manbun dented my car and gave me a fake phone number, promising me he'd pay half of the repair. Every time I would see this dude partying downtown, my fingers started itching around the joystick, my soul yearning to ride the 6 mph, 425 lbs. power wheelchair over that hippie scum piece of shit. I get so mad sometimes at able-bodied a-holes

The truth, of course, is that MDMA may have helped my neuropathic pain, or at least the grief over losing the fight with my body. By the way, how freaking cool is it that me, a Gen X-er, was offered ecstasy at High Mountain Hideout?! A wildly enthusiastic friend ran towards me and said, "Hey Kaatje, do you want some Molly?"

"I don't know Molly, who are you taking about?" I replied.

"Molly, you know. Molly!"

"But I don't know a Molly"

"*Ecstasy*, Kaatje, do you want Ecstasy?"

"God no, I'm already too cheerful!"

At the only European rave I've ever attended, in the 80's, someone offered me a piece of paper with a strawberry, of course I said *no* back then too. However, unbeknownst to me till after he'd swallowed the drug, my brother did not say no. A freelance journalist friend had invited us to the massive rave, he was deeply embedded with creepy Amsterdam folks nicknamed *the Family*—that never ends well, does it? Later he described me in Dutch *Playboy* as "A vision of beauty, like an angel amidst the wild ravers, her long blond hair to her waist, dressed in white, completely fucking sober." Proof that the articles in *Playboy Magazine* do matter—even if I certainly was nothing like my friend described.

Honestly, perhaps I have always been too much of a wuss to experiment, even if the cartels played a role in my abstinence. I'm equally grateful that I never turned to alcohol, aside from that one time in 2016 when I had two, three beers. On top of anti-seizure meds for the neuropathic pain, most likely I was tipsy, and I immediately banged a 26-year-old Mexican-American weed dealer. Mr. Weed Dealer and I had a hilarious conversation in bed.

"My weed is so good, you need sunglasses for the crystals," he bragged.

"That's cute, but I hate weed!"

"Oh. Well, you know you'd get laid way more often if you weren't disabled," he then said, "you're hot. I dated a 42-year-old and she looked older than you."

"Oh you're sweet. Well, we're out of condoms, so that's that," I replied.

"Come one, let me dip it in again, a little. I can tell you are safe."

"No way, I am not *that* drunk!"

Sadly, it turned out that sleeping with weed dealers was no anathema for loneliness, but weirdly, it did give me a little bit of confidence.

* * *

I kept searching for something that would bring my neuropathic pain down to livable levels. I was desperate and had to find a remedy so I could quit writing in documents labeled "My Suicidal Year." I had heard about a compound called DMT (N, N- Dimethyltryptamine) which could help alter one's perception of—and relationship to—pain.[77] A friend and I had gone to Shane Mauss' stand-up comedy at The Box Theater. Shane had shattered both his ankles from a fall while hiking and was left with significant residual pain, he self-medicates with kratom.

Shane's tour was titled "A Good Trip" and he talked about how hard it was to get your hands on DMT, that it was wicked underground. My friend turned to me and whispered, "Oh no, it's not hard to get at all!" She's a Burner, and no matter their website and PR, I quip on stage, "Burning Man's dogma? 'It's all about radical self-reliance and art!' Nah….it's a drug and alcohol-fueled sex rave! Really, should you ever need really good designer drugs, you ought to befriend Burners!"

In all seriousness, I became really interested in the healing possibilities of DMT, after reading Dr. Rick Strassman's book, *DMT: The Spirit Molecule.*[78] Dr. Strassman, while doing research at the University of New Mexico, had safely injected hundreds of people with DMT in the nineties. I learned that

DMT is the psychoactive ingredient in a hallucinogenic plant called ayahuasca, used for spiritual ceremonies in South America. If ayahuasca, solely, is consumed, the stomach digests it too quickly, and the perception-altering visions, and potential medicinal benefits, do not occur.

So, another plant, a vine, is added to prevent too rapid a breakdown of the beneficial molecular components. When prepared correctly, ayahuasca's side effects are prolonged vomiting, and the spiritual ceremony can last up to twelve hours. Since I'm completely incontinent while throwing up, spending a day in my own urine and vomit did not sound like fun, at all.

Smoking DMT instead of ingesting ayahuasca and the vine, seemed a no-brainer. After a bit of begging, my burner friend let me smoke some of hers. It was not very relaxing, though. It felt as if my body disappeared into my hospital bed. Also, my ceiling really tripped me out, but let's face it, even sober, my ceiling looks trippy. Mostly, I was painfully aware of the sounds my antsy friend was making, constantly tapping her shoes on my laminate flooring and flicking her lighter while she chain-smoked.

Sure, I traveled into outer space, while simultaneously seeing a sharp tool pressed against my T4 thoracic (chest level) vertebrae. That hurt! I saw all the neurons in my skull, colorful and exploding beautifully, and the cells that were trying to repair the damage inside T4. I suppose that more spiritual people than I would have explained it as magical. I think it's entirely logical that my mind would take me to T4, where the vascular, benign tumor resides, given my active imagination and my medical background.

For a few weeks after smoking DMT, it seemed my mind and body felt a bit better. Like a cloud had lifted, although that could have been a placebo effect. Against my ethics, and hoping it came from an American laboratory and not the Mexican cartels, I then bought my own DMT. I justified it as an act of rebellion against the FDA, the DEA, and the CDC. For DMT is also a Schedule I drug, just like heroin, LSD, marijuana, and ecstasy. Doesn't it seem incredible that the DEA Controlled Substance Act is this archaic, while more and more states are liberating marijuana? The DEA also seems confused and arbitrarily in its classification system.

This is what the DEA states about oxycodone and cocaine, both Schedule II: "These drugs are considered dangerous, with use potentially leading to severe psychological and physical dependence." Bizarrely, Schedule IV drugs such as Valium (diazepam) and Soma (carisoprodol) are described as, "[…] drugs with a *low* potential for abuse and *low* risk of dependence." Uh, no. Especially the benzodiazepines, which can be incredibly addictive. Subutex (buprenorphine) is classified as Schedule III and is listed as having *less* of an abuse potential than methadone, a Schedule II drug. Both are used for opioid addiction disorders, but one is considered "safer."

Think money could be a motivator? Bingo. When buprenorphine was not generic yet, a special interest group lobbied to have buprenorphine classified as Schedule III, whereas generic methadone stayed Schedule II. This book won't allow to delve deeply into those discrepancies but will be addressed in my next book. According to Lorie Gonzalez et al; "In Florida, the number of carisoprodol-/meprobamate (a metabolite of carisoprodol)-related deaths in 2005 *exceeded those attributed to opioids, including heroin and fentanyl.*"[79]

At a time, when faith in our public institutions is at a historic low, the DEA fails to acknowledge that the so-called safer, Schedule II buprenorphine, is now used for the newest pill mills. Naturally, buprenorphine overdose deaths are on the rise, in the Appalachians. (It is much harder to divert the liquid that is dispensed by methadone clinics, than buprenorphine pills.)

* * *

Buying and smoking DMT was risky, as I knew marginalized people— including the disabled—and minor drug offenders were harshly sentenced. US incarceration sentences seemed completely arbitrary. Every country has a different approach to drugs, but no other country than the US has this high a prison population. Or such long sentences, without decent rehabilitation. Unfortunately, letting everyone get off on drug charges will not have as large an impact as described in the brilliant book *The New Jim Crow*.

Don't get me wrong; African Americans, Hispanics and other minorities are truly suffering under the seemingly vicious, increasingly militarized policing that has become the norm in America—although, who could have predicted the cartels would come to America, armed with machine guns? Exonerating all drug offenders would decrease the prison population by 25%, even so, we would have the largest prison population in the world (but hey, it's a start, let's do it). Regrettably, the misguided War on Drugs, and mandatory sentencing was supported by both black and white politicians, churches and community leaders.

Obtaining my very own DMT for my ex-adrenaline junkie brain was so much fun though. Pretty cool for someone who'd only smoked hash—legally.

Our hash came from Lebanon, Afghanistan and Morocco, not Mexico. Certainly, it involved bloodshed too. Less fun was finding out how to smoke DMT without my Burner friend. It came as a yellow powder and Googling *how to smoke DMT* said the best way to smoke it was with a *crack pipe.* Really? Are you messing with me? Holy moly, I've never even done cocaine, and I've gotta go to Ray's Smoke Shop and ask for a crack pipe? Well.

Me: "Hi! Do you sell crack pipes? It's not for crack."

Antonio, the handsome black clerk looked askew: "You can't say 'crack pipe' in my store."

"That's hilarious. You're joking right, these shady looking pipes and torch lighters are not for crack? I saw those, in Google images!"

"Please, don't say crack. They're bubble pipes." Wow, he sounded so serious.

"Jeez, I've never done *real* drugs, it's for DMT. Have you heard of DMT?"

I did not want Antonio to think of me as a crack addict, as I'd much rather that him and his lovely wife set me up on a blind date with one of their single, older brothers. I smiled extra hard to show him all my teeth. No meth mouth here, Antonio! The irony is that meth mouth is as big a myth as a crack or sad little crack babies. It's not the drug, it's the lifestyle, like skipping on dentist visits, tooth brushing, and lack of healthy food that turns a lovely smile into a meth mouth. Or a baby being born underweight or addicted. I smiled extra hard, to no avail.

"No, and again, don't say crack in my store!"

"Okay. Sorry, it's just, I don't want you to judge me. It's for DMT. Not crack."

Oh my god, the more I tried to suppress "crack," the more I developed crack Tourette's. I finally turned my power wheelchair and looked at weed pipes, no doubt hand blown by underpaid Vietnamese or El Salvadorian children. I couldn't get myself to buy a bubble aka crack pipe, so left Ray's with an ugly ass, fat blue/orange weed pipe that was four times more expensive than a bubble pipe, but what can I say? You think I was kidding? Nope, I'm really an unbelievable wuss sometimes.

* * *

Armed with the hideous, overpriced weed pipe, I went home and checked the bookmarked page "How to smoke DMT." Closing your eyes and meditating a few minutes beforehand was highly recommended. I approached it as a vision quest with a purpose: *why am I in so much pain and what can I do?* With that meditative thought and an optimistic attitude, I grabbed my lighter.

The yellow DMT powder was packed in between trim, the crappy leftovers from weed harvest that won't get anyone high. Except me, as I think trim is way too strong. The DMT had to be heated well, then inhaled deeply. It smells like burned plastic. I laid down on my right side and immediately had an auditory *breakthrough*. Apparently, this is a kind of sound barrier your brain creates, with the vibrations going through my entire skull before I floated out into space.

Ten, fifteen minutes later, the DMT had worn off and I felt my logical brain, and my own *self*, surface again. I was no longer caught up in the seemingly unlimited fractals my own neurons projected from my brain by attended a half dozen Fractal Friday shows, sober, at the Albuquerque Planetarium. Jonathan Wolfe is a hero, teaching kids and adults the beauty of fractals, that were a far cry from the fractals my 1990's computer would calculate. Although I literally *heard* the answer to my question, why this much pain and what should I do, the minute I came to, the answer was lost, locked up again in my brain. Sigh. Now I had all this leftover DMT I didn't know what to do with, so I went into the desert with a brilliant musician buddy, Adam James.

It was supposed to be a healing pilgrimage; soaking in hot springs, relaxing the mind and the body. We'd brought my manual wheelchair, but Ojo Caliente was much harder to maneuver than I'd remembered from previous years, and the drive was too long. Before we reached Ojo, we'd stopped on top of a mesa. We'd opened the trunk of my minivan and lounged in the back. It was really windy though and the clouds were moving fast above us. I was in tears, happy to be back in my beloved, beautiful outdoors, thanks to Adams' driving. In the end, most of the DMT ended up swirling away like yellow clouds, while the rest melted in the metal weed pipe. Adam had brought the wrong kind of pipe!

Overall, buying and smoking DMT seemed a tad stressful, never mind illegal. I also wasn't willing to go under again, just to look for an answer I'd lose on my way out. DMT did elevate my mood for a few weeks, or rather, I felt more normal because my depressive feelings seemed lessened. Yet it did not have a profound or lasting effect on the neuropathic pain. That's a pity, because DMT, at $60 for four doses, is way cheaper than IV ketamine infusions at a private clinic.

PART THREE

First weeklong hospitalization, September 2017

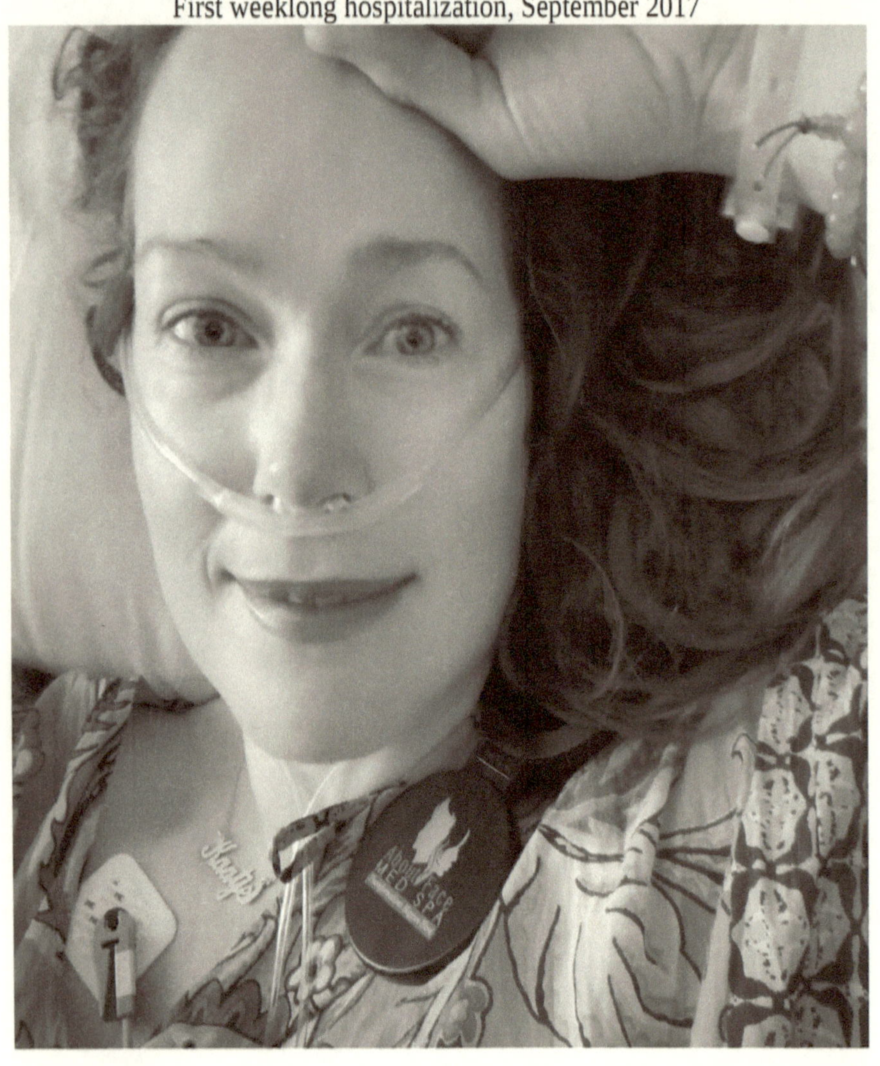

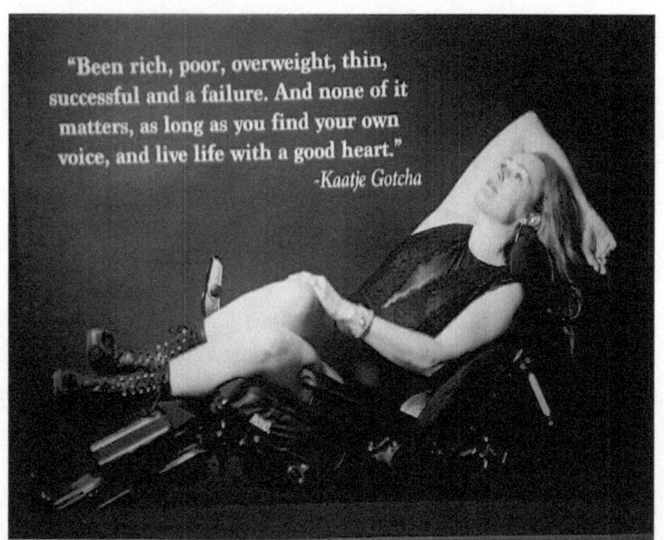

Occupational Therapy Photoshoot by Qiao Qiao Jade
Great set for a sold out show at Aux Dog, yet promoter refuses to pay. Oh, the life of an Albuquerque comic!

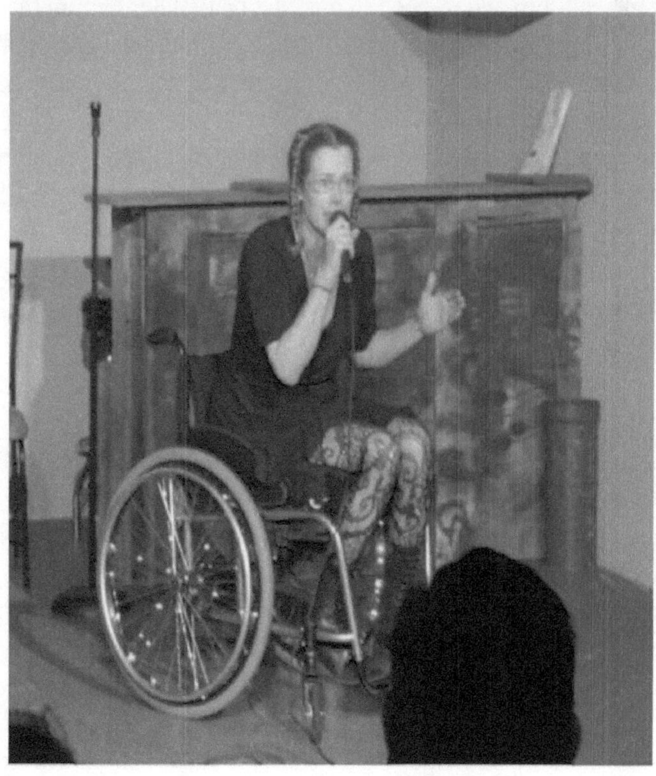

7 "BE CAREFUL OF THE K-HOLE, YO!"

How many 54-year-old quadriplegics are putting albums out? You just have to deal with what you got, try to sustain yourself as best you can, and look to the things you can do. - Curtis Mayfield, musician and tenacious human being

After my haphazard experiments with DMT, and despite all the anti-seizure, anti-muscle spasm, tricyclic antidepressant and opiates, the truth dawned on me that I suffered too much neuropathic pain. And yet, I continued my cautionary approach to opioids: never taking more than one or two 5/325 mg oxycodone IR tablets daily, in addition to the Oxycontin 10 mg ER in the morning and the evening. Gabapentin and baclofen had worked well for the last 12, 13 years.

Dr. Rosenblum from Gaylord Rehab in Connecticut had started me on those very helpful baseline meds. It's just that they were no match against the worsening torment from the adhesive arachnoiditis and the central neuropathic pain syndrome. Over the last two decades I've tried two dozen therapies, sometimes to placate well-meaning friends and strangers—not that it would have proven anything except a testimonial. Correlation is not causation, although with the best of intentions they just wanted to help alleviate my suffering.

Massage therapy, meditation, mindfulness, chanting, craniosacral therapy, cupping, hypnosis, polarity massage, Traditional Chinese Medicine, Reiki, wheelchair, walker, bilateral leg braces, lying down everywhere, anti-gravity boots and inversion therapy, very expensive ASEA healing water, acupuncture, acupressure, myofascial therapy, dry needling, supplements, homeopathy, Cognitive Behavioral Therapy (CBT), physical therapy, trigger point injections, occupational and physical therapy, naturopathy, medical cannabis, epidural steroidal injections, spiritual and esoteric medicine, sexual healing—just kidding, although sex is healthy—prayer, DMT, chiropractic care and CBD oil. To no avail. Maybe I should've tried that Oprah-recommended gratitude journal.

I'm not a huge fan of alternative medicine, those treatments lack robust data, but at least most seem to do no physical harm except to my wallet. And it is nice to receive a massage in a room with a heated blanket, a little fountain and soothing New Age music. I'm reminded of that New Mexico teacher, the one who self-medicates with a small dose of psilocybin every few months to stave off her cluster, aka 'suicide' headaches.

Because psilocybin is a Scheduled I drug—recall, lumped into the same category as LSD, marijuana and heroin—research has been incredibly difficult. Despite small, recent advances through MAPS research and cannabis legalization, it may be another decade before new guidelines and deregulation pave the way for a saner approach to psychotherapeutic medications and treatment. I swear, a thousand years from now, people will look back at this era of pain medicine and call it The Second Middle Ages.

The political/medical/health insurance system regularly denies treatments that are superior, such as a multi-disciplinary approach to complex pain and/or psychiatric disorders. Adequate preventative medical care and pain relief, combined with an emphasis on helping patients cope emotionally and mentally with their chronic conditions—addressing issues like isolation and despair, is what we need badly. If our government's focus were to change in the arenas of mental health, perhaps more suicides could be prevented too.

Globally, one million people kill themselves every year; it's the second leading cause of death for 15 to 29-year-olds.[80] The financial cost of US psychiatric disorders are astronomical: $89 billion for non-institutionalized care, and another $193 billion in lost productivity and half of the prison population has a mental health problem.[81] The USA could be the greatest hope for mankind, if they were willing to embrace and fund more medical research on therapeutic psilocybin, LSD, MDMA, and ketamine—recall those substances may alleviate alcohol use disorder, PTSD and depression.

Even if extensive research shows those compounds have few to no medical benefits, those studies could determine they pose little harm for recreational users. At least then we would know, and quite possibly, we could start re-classifying drugs in the Controlled Substance Act.

* * *

So, still desperate to find some relief for the worsening neuropathy and not finding it in the American medical system, in 2015 I'd reached out to my

Dutch pain specialist to see if he would admit me for ketamine infusion, shown on the hospital's website. Recall, ketamine is a so-called dissociative anesthetic and listed as a World Health Organization *essential medicine* for its' high safety profile. Ketamine doesn't depress breathing, like other anesthetic medication, so can be applied in countries or battlefields where electricity is intermittent.

It is used for childbirth and appendectomy, and even in some forward-thinking American ERs for severe, acute ache like that of complicated fractures, or injuries, especially in a pediatric setting. As for the much-hyped reputation of ketamine as a party drug: "The WHO Committee concluded that ketamine abuse does *not* pose a global public health threat, while controlling it could limit access to the only anaesthetic and pain killer available in large areas of the developing world." By now, I'm gung-ho for the WHO.[82]

How safe is ketamine? Of 70,000 reviewed anesthesia cases, there was one fatality, and this was mostly because of the patients' complex comorbidities, according to research by Strayer & Nelson. Their conclusion? "Reports of significant cardiorespiratory adverse events are rare, despite ketamine's frequent use in austere, poorly monitored settings. Dysphoric emergence phenomena occur in 10% to 20% of cases; sedating medications are effective in preventing and managing these reactions."[83]

The Dutch physician literally scoffed at my suggestion to try ketamine, although truly 'twas more a desperate plea than a suggestion, at this point. Ketamine treatment is on the hospitals' website! Ironically, until this gnarly encounter, I had not yet known what scoffing sounded like but there it was: damn those were some ugly ass noises. So, despite the inpatient ketamine treatment offered by his Pain Management team, and his diagnosis of central neuropathic pain syndrome—brought on by the intramedullary spinal cord lesion at T4 chest level—he looked dumbfounded. Central neuropathic pain, just like adhesive arachnoiditis leads to, no surprise there, intractable and incurable neuropathic torment. To make his point, he scoffed *again*, then scolded me.

"We're still far away from ketamine treatment, you have a few options left. Besides, ketamine has a lot of side effects," my Dutch doctor, the King in his Ivory Tower, said to this lowly peasant.

Or was it serf, or plebe? Yeah, he talked to me like I was a serf. The Ivory Tower is what the Dutch call the patriarchal, authoritarian attitude by doctors, who believe they're always right and the patient is always wrong. I wished

I'd said, *"Side effects? You know what undertreated neuropathy's side effect is? Suicide, Dr. Dipshit."*

Instead of allowing me to try ketamine therapy, he increased the amitriptyline dose and prescribed a TENS unit. I tried the TENS unit for three months, placing patches above and below T4—no small feat—but it only increased back spasms. I kept swimming in the nearby heated pool, with added physical therapy exercises and stretches in the adjacent hot tub. And yet, it was not enough. The amitriptyline at 150 mg daily he'd prescribed provoked such dry mouth, I had to quickly drop back to a 75 mg nightly dose.

* * *

Talking on-line with other patients suffering from severe agony showed me that I'm not the only one who gets treated poorly. Every penny seems to go to the people at the top driving the policy and system-wide decisions, which ultimately results in the marginalization of more and more patients. Meanwhile, they shave their budgets on the backs of our anguish. The politicians keep living the good life with favorable health insurance, a car with a chauffeur, catered meals, and promises of a cushy job after they leave politics. I'm reminded of Mark Twain, "Suppose you were an idiot. And suppose you were a member of Congress. But I repeat myself."

Why is it, that one in three Medicare patients has surgery, one year before their death—and 8% in the week before they die? Does that sound like that is in the best interest of the patient, or is the patients' insurance milked for money, quality of life be damned, business as usual?[84] Medical and pharmaceutical companies lobby the government and health insurance companies to reimburse back surgeries and other procedures, some of which trigger even more physical discomfort.

Medicare abuse is rampant: research after research finds that 10-20% of surgeries aren't medically necessary.[85] Can't blame it all on nefarious organizations or individuals though. Americans want, no, demand aggressive interventions, even if for example, their geriatric loved one is on a ventilator. Heroic measures at that age aren't pretty, and American citizens deserve compassionate, honest and realistic conversations by the medical teams. And for mainstream media to tell the truth on those horrifying, trauma-inducing deaths, instead of a more humanistic palliative or hospice care.

Policy makers are culpable though. Especially since the CDC Opioid Guidelines came out, they have pushed epidural steroidal injection treatments onto patients. In 2014 the FDA send out a warning letter stating corticosteroids ought not be injected in the epidural space. They stopped at forbidding it outright, which would have exposed the FDA, the pharmaceutical industry and medical providers to lawsuits. After my trusted primary care provider was forced to stop prescribing opioids, I tried setting up an appointment with the three pain clinics in my town, which has a metropolitan population of 900,000 souls. None of them accepted patients for medication management, all were interventional only, offering epidural steroidal injections at $2-3000 a pop.

And so, instead of reimbursing psychotherapy, functional medicine—a multimodal approach that includes Physical Therapy and Cognitive Behavioral Therapy—and ketamine treatments, our bodies are burning with iatrogenic afflictions, perhaps generated by ineffectual treatments, or botched lumbar punctures, back surgeries or childbirth epidurals. Recall that severe neuropathic pain that goes untreated or undertreated can quickly progress to central sensitization. Once my Dutch doctor proclaimed a hard *no* to the in-hospital ketamine therapy, that left me searching for answers in America, again. Rather than kill myself, I realized I wanted to whatever it takes to continue living, even in this defunct body.

* * *

When I began learning about ketamine in earnest, I had already started open mics and comedy showcases. I was happy to channel my creative energy in order to offset the horror show of my daily, increasingly bedridden existence. I sincerely wished they hadn't phoned the trauma helicopter and couldn't decide whether it was a blessing or a curse that I was alive. But I leaned towards *hey, this is my reality* even if it seemed an unbearable fate. By now, with documents titled, "My Super Suicidal Year," it was clear that, if I did not do something to change, I wouldn't exist for much longer as an organism.

I had learned through Googling that ketamine might provide relief for those with chronic neuropathic pain, CRPS, other neuropathies, and phantom limb pain. So, I browsed online and called clinics. I soon found out ketamine infusions are expensive. A vial of the drug is only $30, but clinics need professional staff trained to administer it and help patients cope with the side effects. There was the overhead, and of course, good malpractice insurance to consider.

Treatment prices varied widely. A Los Angeles clinic charged $1800 for a four-hour ketamine infusion; Portland, $2500; Denver, $825; Cardiff Clinic in California, $700; and the Ketamine Wellness Center in Mesa, Arizona, $750. I decided on the Mesa clinic for several reasons: their professionalism, courteous attitude, pricing and *private* treatment rooms. During treatment, a provider sits next to you for safety and monitoring. Most importantly, it was a six-hour drive from Albuquerque. I sold my minivan to pay for the medical treatments, as I now lived downtown and use my power wheelchair to go to the gym and comedy open mics.

I told myself it wasn't a huge deal, but that's not true. I cried about losing one more tool of independence. I comforted myself with practical reasoning: no more maintenance, parking, and insurance. Besides, driving by myself wasn't fun anymore, with the lumbosacral burning and the gnawing sensations worsening after as little as five to ten minutes, on top of the leg and trunk hypersensitivity. Even the pressure of the seat belt hurt. I'd fainted while driving in March of 2016, a combination of dehydration and anti-seizure medications, which had resulted in a $900 repair bill.

Selling the car was a no-brainer, but it also meant I had no way to escape this town and start over—which had been my coping strategy for most of my life. I was literally stuck and needed to be okay with that. The Ketamine Wellness Center near Phoenix recommended a series of three infusions, one per day for three days. Aside from affordability, the clinic seemed medially professional with their review of my case. I was interviewed by a psychologist via a secure video conference website and filled out psych eval after eval. One of the hundreds of personality questions was, "Do you believe you'd make a good comedian?" Yup.

Unbeknownst to me, all throughout 2016 my mom and sister had been extremely worried about my physical and mental state. While I was coordinating with the Ketamine Wellness Center and making car and hotel reservations, Nicolien flew in from the Netherlands, for the first time in since becoming a doting mom in 2008. Amazingly, she had historic ties to Phoenix, it's where she interned for her Bachelors in Tourism degree from January 1992 through July 1993.

As a little girl, and even as a teenager, she studied hard with the goal of opening her own tearoom and restaurant business. Nicolien had been over the moon scoring a coveted spot in the United States. Unfortunately, since Nicolien had been stationed at the Phoenician Resort in October 1992, she was the first of my family to get the dreaded call I was fighting for my life in Riverside General. (My parents were out of reach in that pre-cell phone, pre-internet era, after visiting Nicolien they had just reached the Colorado River inside the Grand Canyon.

This time, during another New Mexican winter, my body smarting even more from the cold, she would drive me to Arizona in our rented minivan. Despite our challenging relationship, I realized how much I loved her. Although that could have been the 2.5 mg of oxycodone that kicked in while we were heading to our hotel in Mesa. Nicolien, now with a bachelor's in nursing degree and over a decade of experience, was in the room with me during my first ketamine treatment on January 9th, 2017.

* * *

Nurse Tiffany started the IV around 9:15 a.m., and then Jonathan, the PA-C, started the first loading dose of ketamine—65 mg. At first, I was completely comfy, it was like flying business class as a teenager to modeling jobs, the few times I'd lucked out. I had two blankets and was seated in what seemed, at the beginning, a comfortable lounger. The private room was standard chic with that generic art. A flower reproduction, the kind of art my talented mom loathed, as people seemed to want posters instead of real paintings, even if they were priced affordably. Have I already mentioned my mom is an outstanding fine artist?

I floated away, while Tiffany played a stand-up comedy special by Jen Kirkman, per my request. I felt spacey. I recalled, again, loving feelings towards my sister. I thought, ketamine is the bomb, my agony feels different already. I made a mental note that, after the treatment, Nicolien and I should visit Ikea to return some online purchases and eat at the Ikea restaurant. I was trying to write some comedy jokes for my next gig when I quickly found out it was hard, typing in Google Docs on my smartphone with a ketamine drip running. I was writing obsessive—and repetitive—notes:

I'm on ketamine now and it feels as I'm floating. Tiffany the nurse grew up in Gallup. I'm playing my favorite SoundCloud list. I feel great. Okay I've been on ketamine for an hour now. This shit's strong. I'm an independent entity, yet Dr. Susan Blackmore comes to mind. I'm not in control of my life. Should not have eaten two waffles this morning. Live and learn. Note to self: Don't eat two waffles right before your ketamine treatment. I have no idea how I'm holding this smartphone on ketamine. Just some tips: no waffles before ketamine. Will be here 'til 1:40 p.m., Tiffany says the adrenaline overcomes the fear when you're skydiving. Yeah, can't say I like ketamine.

Again, thank goodness for all the fractal shows in the Albuquerque Planetarium because this was EXACTLY like being inside a fractal, floating through galaxies and careening through space and time, back to before the birth of the Universe, feeling as if I'm a molecule inside the civilizations I saw rise and fall as the ketamine dosage increased. Uh-oh, I don't feel so good now, is this what Derek meant by when he said: "Be careful of the K-hole, yo!" He'd warned me, said that when he snorts ketamine recreationally, he uses an equal amount of ketamine, ecstasy and cocaine. Boy, that just sounded dangerous, and expensive. Derek called it "doing party lines." I sure have interesting friends. Uh-oh, I, my own self is gone. I think I died. I'm positive I'm going to die.

Aside from the silly and introspective observations, within seconds, the ketamine decreased the severe, chest level neuropathy as well as the agony of the lumbosacral adhesive arachnoiditis. The worst of the excruciating sensations, the allodynia, had seemed to calm down. I was no longer aware of the pressure of my clothes. That feeling of someone pouring molten lead inside my spinal cord and body had decreased by at least 90 percent. It was as if a firefighter, a very cute one, had finally put out the bonfire raging inside my body. Gentle, cold streams had replaced the fire like, burning feelings below the chest and waist.

***

Nicolien, who'd become an accomplished nurse after my accident, shifted in her chair and suddenly, I strongly sensed her presence. She's younger by a year and a half, and seems adamantly against recreational drugs, even those that may help in a therapeutic setting such as MDMA and psilocybin. My wonderful, smart sister with the big, generous heart has battled dysthymia for three decades, and yet it seems there's nothing I can do to help alleviate her suffering, just like she can't modulate mine.

At any rate, knowing my sister's stance, and being the oldest, I didn't even want to worry her by asking for Versed (a benzodiazepine and anti-anxiety medication), or Phenergan (nausea medication), both of which can dull the hallucinatory effects while concurrently causing drowsiness. I didn't think it was appropriate to bring up the fact I was finally *tripping balls* and not enjoying it one bit. Then I thought, *Mind over matter*. She won't notice. Hah! Mind over matter worked in mountaineering, but not with this infusion.

It was as if I was drowning, and dying with every breath, just like "The OA" protagonist in Season One of the Netflix series. I had horrible hallucinations, but the pain-squelching effects were immediate and life-altering. When the infusion was done, feeling emotionally and physically drained as if I'd nearly succumbed to the water's pull, it seemed I managed to crawl back onto a beach, inside the safety of my own consciousness once again. We picked up my Diet Rockstar that Chera had kept cold—which would become my go-to after infusion treat—ate a few cookies and left the clinic. We drove straight to Tempe's Ikea to return some stuff and eat Swedish food.

I loved that Tempe location; the beautiful palm trees out front along the road framing the building, which was really a museum and testament for great design. We did get stuck inside a monumental, inescapable *Ikea-hole* though, when we struggled to find the nearest exit from the Market Place. The morning after my first infusion felt miraculous. The nearby Days Hotel had a heated, outdoor pool and I swam for thirty minutes. For the first time in over a decade, I moved through the water without the gnawing, gut-wrenching sensations that felt as if my left leg was being attacked by a shark.

Even my sacral ache was negligible. I could walk a bit more, despite the bilateral lower leg atrophy. Sitting in my wheelchair was a little more tolerable, as well. And perhaps the biggest added benefit was that my suicidal feelings and desperate thoughts were gone. Poof. Yet, the hallucinations on the first day had been intolerable, that comfortable-seeming chair way too painful after three hours, it had worsened my sacral anguish. I had my mind made up to *not* return for the second infusion. Nicolien encouraged me to email the clinic, a few hours after the infusion. She wanted me to try at least a second infusion.

The Ketamine Wellness Center was immediately responsive. Chera ensured me I'd have a different treatment room with a much more padded La-Z-Boy-type lounger. It turned out the chair they put me in during my first treatment was normally used for psychiatric infusion treatment, which typically only last for 45 minutes. Because I could not yet put the ketamine infusion and the psychoactive side effects into perspective, I threw the baby out with the bathwater and asked for a different nurse, or medic, altogether.

Poor Tiffany, whom I blamed for my awful side effects, when it was I who was too stubborn to ask for ameliorating medications. By infusion number three, I had wizened up, send my sister to Target to have fun and buy gifts for her two young kids, and said to the attending nurse: "Hit me, with *everything* you've got!"

* * *

Those first few infusions were always the same: I felt my consciousness slip, my entire being, my personhood, becoming unhinged, saw myself as a molecule drifting in space. Often, I wasn't even a passenger in a galactic-looking spaceship, but instead, was part of the insulation material of the ship, a kind of dark foam that shapeshifted all the time. It was kind of exhausting, and fear permeated my every cell and pore. On ketamine, my ruminative and obsessive self—or whatever was left of it—pondered why I always ended up in the engine room, instead of being cool and part of the crew. I longed to be on the bridge of the Battlestar Galactica with Dee and Captain Adama.

But, stuck in that engine room, I wasn't even a hammer or wrench; I was a molecule, a neuron, a proton or quark. Small. I saw myself as so small. Again, I wished I would have seriously *tripped balls* recreationally sometime in my past, instead of those higgledy-piggledy attempts with DMT. Next to ketamine, DMT seemed like a walk in the park. My sense of self usually completely disappeared, and I hated it. I shouldn't have, because my rational mind knows that I construct my own reality, or rather that 'Free will is an illusion.' Dr. Susan Blackmore studies free will, she theorizes we all feel as if there is continuity to the 'self,' a consistency of being, such as believing our personalities are real, for example.[86]

It is not just Blackmore who talks about this concept. Other scholars such as Bruce Hood and David Hume have also concluded there is no self; it is a construct, an illusion.[87] The self is a powerful, narrative arc that our brain creates. In the words of Bruce Hood: "We know that if you alter the physical state of the brain through a head injury, dementia or drugs, each of these *changes our self.* Whether it is through damage, disease or debauchery, we know that the self must be the output of the material brain."

I remain in awe of one of our greatest illusions, our vision. We are not aware that the world we witness enters our retinas upside down. The brain turns this image 180 degrees, so we see a table on the floor, in alignment with gravity.[88] The fact the brain constructed that powerful illusion means we should not underestimate the brain's ability to fool us when it comes to ourselves. We may not exist the way we think we exist, in the sense that our selves are carefully constructed, every day, anew.

Strangely, the ketamine visions brought me closer to my dad, who is a big fan of philosopher Daniel Dennett. Dennett opined there are only mental processes, the brain holds no location for a self. Ketamine opened my mind to these kinds of realizations. It challenged me to reconcile my knowledge of science and philosophy with my hallucinatory, mystical visions. Some of my subsequent visions were hilarious. I don't know which was worse, finding out that I am *the* gatekeeper for the entirety of existence, or feeling as though, if I fell deeper into the event horizon, I would surely die.

And of course, as the gatekeeper of the Universe, my visions told me I had to abide by just one minor condition to prevent total annihilation of mankind, and that was to *never* break up with my boyfriend. To my surprise even a born again, hardcore atheist like myself had a brain that created a justifiable existence in this Universe, with specific rules and regulations, just like with any other religion. I say born again because, although I was raised in an atheist cult—my family—I got sidetracked for about a decade by Carlos Castaneda and others who were either visionaries, or charlatans. Being on ketamine, therefore, confirmed to me that all religions are based on our brain's faulty premises.

When one has found *the* truth, only *if*—and yes, there is always an if— one is duty-bound to abide by at least one or, perhaps, many more stipulations. Like prayer, or believing that taking extremely high, unsafe doses of vitamins will cure you of anything—I'm scolding you, Dr. Weil for perpetuating Dr Linus Pauling's Vitamin C myth. If humanity is viewed as a species hardwired to hold magical beliefs, then perhaps society will become easier to accept and understand, to me. From orthorexia—the belief that eating only healthy, GMO-free foods are acceptable—to religions, or cults, our brains demand a framework to explain reality. How does such thinking arise? It's because we are pattern-seeking organisms. We should all be taught from birth that correlation is not causation.

This great mystical vision I experienced under the influence of ketamine told me that my Navajo beau and I had to keep banging each other. Exclusively. If we didn't, the entire space-time continuum would become unraveled and humanity would be doomed. I've gotta admit, it's kind of hard to remain an atheist when your brain is bathing in ketamine and you feel like you and your lover are responsible for humanity's salvation, or its demise. The ketamine experience confirmed for me that all brains—even mine—are hardwired for esoteric, supernatural thinking. It had to be, because the alternative, that mysticism is real would have meant an annihilation of my rational beliefs.

* * *

The traumatic event horizon experience during my very first infusion was completely of my own making though. It really *was* my fault being stuck right there at the edge, trying to avoid falling into a black hole. Not only did I refuse all meds for sedation, ten minutes prior to the treatment, in the waiting room I'd read a *New Scientist* article featuring Stephen Hawking's revised theory on black holes. Classic, rookie mistake: do not read astrophysics just before your very first ketamine infusion! Especially about black holes and event horizons.

Because I didn't have time to read all the way through the article before the treatment, I missed the essential last paragraph, where Dr. Hawking says something to the effect of: "Do not despair if you ever get stuck in a black hole. Maybe information does come through in another universe." *What?! And why couldn't the article have started off with that statement, instead of a blurb about Stephen Hawking's revolutionary revised treatise on black holes?*[89]

Wait, has Stephen Hawking himself tried DMT and ketamine? And if so, would we be okay with that? Perhaps *that* would finally take the stigma off psychedelics. Dr. Hawking has traveled a lot and seemed to have friends and admirers all over the world, so it's not inconceivable that he might have had Burning Man buddies.

To me, at this point the only downside to ketamine treatment were indeed the side effects of hallucinations, vivid dreams, and visions. Well, in that case I accept the side-effects wholeheartedly, since the pain relief of ketamine is simply unmatched with any other medications out there.

Weirdly, before doing ketamine infusions, I had not been able to sleep on my left side. Yet immediately after the first treatment my body wanted to lie on the left side, as if it yearned to make up for 15, 20 years of sleeping on the right side only. That was an unexpected, and delightful outcome.

For us sisters, despite our challenging relationship, it had been a very special time in Arizona. I found relief from my ordeal and lifelong pain sentence, and Nicolien had even hiked to the top of her beloved Camelback Mountain. She was now eager to return to her kids, and after a tearful and loving goodbye in Albuquerque, she disappeared into the airport for the 18-hour journey.

I was ready for a future that would surely be filled with nothing but happiness, comedy, and writing.

8 YOU WILL NEVER EAT A BURRITO IN THIS TOWN AGAIN

Comedy is lonely, vicious and cruel. - Will Ferrell, comedic genius

Sounds like Will Ferrell never had to run away from an avalanche, or hike while being hungry! I must admit, even after all these years, heck, after two and a half decades, mountaineering is in my blood. Aged six, I had been hiking and climbing for years, and had already scaled the Triglav, Yugoslavia's highest mountain peak. Before my accident it was the only life I had ever known. It is a simple life, too.

You make do. You suffer. You keep hiking despite blisters filled with blood, through wild, cold Alpine rivers and glacier runoff, whose waters would soothe your feet and replenish water bottles. Your parents use thin plastic bags to cover your socks, but there is so much water, snow, and sweat, at the end of the day, you don't know what soaked your feet.

You seek shelter and improvise your rations, so an evening meal might be mashed potatoes from powder, mixed with dried kale—known in Holland as *farmer's cabbage*—and dried shrimps for protein. You will recall it as one of the best meals you ever had, while huddling inside a small, primitive stone shack placed on the route to two mountain cabins, each another four, five six hour walk you cannot reach. Night fell fast, high in the Julian Alps.

You will climb into caves with your dad, after conquering a 45-degree sloped snow field covered with a layer of ice, and the caves high up have an abundance of crystal. You will hack off some and take it home; decades later the crystals remain in a jar on your nightstand. You will solo hike the Jalovec mountain with your dad, who bursts out crying on the top, and you won't know how to console him. You will run and scream from aggressive horse flies biting and chasing you and your family down a Spanish mountain side.

You will break into abandoned ski buildings, and shiver inside the sleeping bag you carry on your small nine-year-old frame. Your father will steal chips as a treat, and necessary calories as they greatly underestimate the nourishment needs of young children. You will beg for food. You learn to look sad and pathetic, so that the few fellow mountaineers you encounter on a snowfield or a steep path take pity and give you salami, cheese, nuts, and chocolate. And after all that hustling, you had to fight your folks, who would've killed for a treat, too.

You witness the corpse of a dead teen, taken to a shed. You put yellow mountain flowers by the door. You know it is your fault your family had to live through this, and it will haunt you. You know the dead climber will become another small memorial, an oval-shaped souvenir of a short life once lived, usually with a little cross above it. In fact, you can't climb a mountain without following a trail of those sad souvenirs, such as *Paulina Dragic, 1955-1974.*

Your mountains, conquered with perseverance, tenacity and with the understanding that once you would be back in the valleys, there was a supermarket with actual food for sale. These are the happiest years of your life, and when life in the cities bored you, and you were unhappy or had another conflict with a photographer, you escaped to the mountains. Alone, with a small tent, or a piece of plastic.

You will sleep on a mountain ledge in the Catskills, and after another breathtaking morning hike, you arrived for brunch at your Ford Modeling agent's weekend home, your dad's old altimeter around your neck. You didn't know supermodel Elle McPherson was going to be there, and her gnarly, old photographer husband, Gilles Bensimon. You were embarrassed about your smell and your unkempt appearance, and disappeared again, on another solo hike, or took a dangerous riverboat into the Amazonas, never bothering with yellow fever or other vaccines.

You were the clown, the silly one cheering up your siblings and parents, when you had to outrun a snow avalanche in the French Alps, or when you got lost, even if you were exhausted or close to tears yourself. You made your siblings laugh so hard, milk exploded through their nostrils. Your biggest treat was going to Peter Sellers' Pink Panther and James Bond movies in a real movie theater, and later, got mightily confused by the movie *Being There.* What the heck was Shirley MacLaine doing to that bedpost?

* * *

It is another October, decades after being a small child and teenager.

Another anniversary of the skydiving accident. For some reason, the weeks surrounding the anniversary of my survival—that's how I've come to think of it—always seem full of life-changing events. October of 2016 was no exception. By this point, I needed comedy like I needed air. It was the only creative outlet that truly connected my heart to the outside world and made me forget about the torment for a few minutes.

Between August 2015 and August 2016, I performed at 106 open mics and showcases, despite that 12-day stay at Lovelace rehabilitation hospital in November/December 2015. For many weeks, I wasn't able to make it out, and there wasn't one venue where I did not have to lie down, to alleviate the throbbing sacrum and the shooting neuropathy from chest to toes. It was a physical hell, even with an available couch or a booth. Most of the time I couldn't use my power wheelchair: Sun Van, the accessible public van, did not allow for comics' late—and chaotic—hours. Besides, Sun Van's shocks hurt my spine more.

So, when I had another unpaid gig, at a Comic Con, I schlepped all the requirements to make myself somewhat comfortable; camping mat, Moroccan blanket, earplugs, mp3 player loaded with mindfulness recording, backpack, meds, Hot Toes, an icepack for my sacrum, in case my pain levels skyrocketed before going on stage. And skyrocket they did, every single time. I created my usual makeshift bed and had rested for twenty minutes, but the *green room* was cold, crowded and had loud music, which always worsened my physical agony. Surrounded by people enjoying their weed pipes and alcohol, I employed plan B—adrenaline—to take my mind of the escalating torment. To each their own, right?

Another comic pushed my wheelchair downstairs, I was keen to attend the advertised speed dating at the event—a week before meeting Dylan—cuz, bro, do *you* know how hard it is to date from your hospital bed? The entry fee was waived for performers, but the promoters hadn't added my name to the guest list. Ticket Girl would not accept my picture and name on the comedy poster as proof I was a performer. Perhaps, I asked, could I please pay now, and for Ticket Girl to return the money to me afterwards? "No."

I asked Ticket Girl if she could—again, *please*—let me in and clear with the manager/organizer after the speed dating event, which started in a few minutes. No matter what solution I came up with, she refused. While waiting for the promoter, sitting upright was no longer feasible. I tucked myself behind my manual wheelchair for a few minutes, trying to get relief for the burning sacral ache, out of the way from the few other people in line. The event wasn't well attended.

Ticket Girl started yelling at me, and I explained the need to decompress my spine. It was cold in the lobby and there was marble flooring, so lying on carpet near the ticket booth seemed the best option. The comedy promoter finally showed up, and said "We've forgotten to update the list, she was supposed to be Rusty Rutherford. Can she enter now?" To which Ticket Girl replied "No." My discomfort was a tiny bit improved and I got back in the wheelchair. At this point, I started disliking Ticket Girl, very, very much.

Out of the blue, the promoter's very intoxicated friend threw down the $35 entry fee and raced my wheelchair through the hallway. When I put my hands on the wheels to slow us down—to avoid clipping people's heels—I was told, "Do that again and I will beat you!" Finally, relief. Glad to be rid of the kidnapping drunk, I leaned on my right hip, threw my defunct legs to an extra chair on my left and was immediately baptized Ms. Hot Wheels by the jovial speed dating host. The fun lasted five minutes, then the promoter yanked me out of the speed dating event and told me I was *banned* from Comic Con.

Be that as it may, the comedy promoters told me I was still allowed to cheer on my fellow comedians, so I made the best of it. I upped my pain meds and crawled into a gold dress with my funky, black orthopedic boots, and a sequin cape. I supported the event by filming a comic who needed footage, then wheeled myself near the stage to ensure the headliner spoke louder, as no one could hear the comic over the bar noise.

As if I wasn't punished enough by being banned, the promoter posted messages across comedy Facebook groups; "Never book Kaatje for an event, she's the most unprofessional comic I've ever worked with. She obstructed the ticket booth. She didn't seem to be in pain." Nonsense. I didn't even bother defending myself. A few weeks later, my reputation destroyed, the promoter came up to me—when my beau and I attended a comedy event— and said; "You know that wasn't personal, right?"

For outsiders who don't understand what it's like to have adhesive arachnoiditis or live a bedridden life, or have seen me in bed, crying from my strange nerve disease and affliction, it's hard to understand why I do not look like a grumpy gimpy. I did explain my dire physical situation at the event— while lying on the floor—but the damage was done. I even offered to write the Comic Con organizer a letter of apology but was told "That won't be allowed."

* * *

Four months later, in February 2017, after five outpatient ketamine infusions, and that winter's worth of turmoil, my physical torment had decreased enough to occasionally venture out to nearby open mics, with my 400 lbs. power wheelchair. One evening my boyfriend Dylan and I headed to one of my regular venues on Central Avenue. We always had so much fun, walking hand in hand despite my big power wheelchair. Of course, I still felt shaken up, but I sorely missed connecting with an audience. It wasn't as if I had a choice either; I needed to feel a sense of purpose in an otherwise bedridden, isolated, and marginalized life.

I asked the hosts if I could—please—be one of the first six comedians in the lineup. Because, despite the ketamine treatments, a 34k wheelchair with specialized settings and a $500 ROHO wheelchair pillow, the fact remained that sitting was agony. The wheelchair pillow was on top of a metal seat. There was no other way to construct it, but it was hardly a sofa with springs, nor a hospital bed. Even the *zero-gravity* wheelchair setting didn't give as much relief as lying horizontally, on my right side.

Throughout the summer of 2016, most hosts had honored my request. But that was before being ostracized from the comedy community. Physically, I couldn't handle any open mic, as most of the time is spent waiting for the show to start, though that was something I did not want to admit. Environmental control became harder and harder. Even if it was warm outside, I had to lie under a blanket because any air-conditioning was always too cold. And in the winter, the heating was never enough.

My body's thermostat seemed permanently wrecked; the buttocks, lower legs, and feet wouldn't stay warm without an outside source of heat. Since I'd started in August 2015 my strategy had been to arrive promptly, hoping to get an early timeslot and get back to my hospital bed as soon as possible. Dylan and I were the first to arrive around 7 p.m., but the host handed the signup sheet to others across the room, who got there much later than I. He finally came around, and I signed up.

"You'll be number 11," the host said, after he'd created the line-up.

"Can I please go earlier?" I asked, again, my voice betraying the whimpering of a hurt animal, with its left leg caught in an iron trap. *Should've been an animal because I would have been put out of my misery by any veterinarian.* Sigh. I never wished so badly that Bad Spot Bill hadn't called that trauma helicopter. *What a waste of a life, being here, begging.* Yes, I do tend to catastrophize when I can't think straight, due to the physical suffering, or a flare up. Nonetheless, I just had to perform, despite my discomfort.

"Everyone wants to go earlier, but some people really need to get out of here," the host shrugged. I thought, *Really?* I'd seen the names of the earlier comics on the line up list knew most of them drank 'til last call, followed by getting high on the patio or in their cars. Not that there was anything wrong with hotboxing, as a Libertarian I don't care what you do as long as you don't hurt anyone. But obviously, this dude was hurting me.

"Look, I'm in so much physical torment. Who else on that list has fallen out of an airplane?" I finally said.

"I know of at least one other person," he shrugged, while turning his back to me, walking away. *Wow, how fucking petty can one person be?* This was an open mic that already started really late, around 8:45 or 9, so meant a future with much agony by the time I could perform six minutes of new and old material. But my set was written, and my mind unwilling to succumb to my physical circumstances.

* * *

I was at a loss to understand how these comics/hosts suddenly seemed so cold and heartless. Some had given me great advice early on, these were people I emulated and saw as mentors, and yet their behavior had inexplicably and drastically changed. It dawned on me that even before being banned from the event, there had been signs that all was not well. By the end of Summer 2016, one of the open mic hosts announced every comic with an awesome introduction, except for me.

Every week, he'd just breathe monotonously into the mic, "Hey this is Kaatje, gotta pee," then shoved the mic in my hand, without a handshake. Unfortunately, I sucked at improvisation, at riffing. That thing Americans do so well! So instead of saying, *"Yay, give it up for our host, even if he has the bladder of a little girl,"* I was flabbergasted.

Despite my disability expertise, I was struggling with my personal, changing physique. I hadn't yet figured out how to manage my manual or power wheelchair in spaces that were not accessible, and the mic cords somehow always ended up twisted around my wheels. Until now, I lacked confidence and was continually flustered before I even started my set. Yet I had never given up on comedy: those moments where it worked, comfortable in myself and my material, were magical. People were laughing at my shit!

Set lists those days read: *Type A Gimpy, spanking, Sprouts, geriatric candy, Muslim hell, Oprah, Deepak Choprah wisdom generator, Tinderstalker, nationalities fucked-23, manscaping, Tinderstalker, crippled comedy tour, baby boomer ass sweat.* I had already filled two hardcover college notebooks with jokes and prepared as if I was taking New Mexico Tech exams. Had to, couldn't deviate or improvise that was a problem. I wrote all jokes out before a set, even an open mic, then made a set list, rehearsed, then gave it my all. For showcases I worked even harder.

Yet no matter where I was performing, the hosts would put someone on stage seconds before it was my turn to go. I'd be ready, with my notebook on my lap, power wheelchair moving toward the mic, when suddenly, someone else was announced. They did this without a courtesy heads up, but I am hardly alone in that respect. This happens to all comedians, everywhere, although I did not see it at the time. I'm a big fan of *sign up is line up* or, whatever spot you sign your name next to is what you get.

Sure enough, that evening one of the hosts refused to let go of the mic when it finally was my turn and did an entire drunken set before me. Technically, that made me number twelve. There went three and a half more agonizing hours of my life, all to perform for a few minutes. I ignored my body's screams and did a quality set by entertaining the entire audience. No one, not even Dylan and a comedy friend, noticed how much I smarted. The evening wasn't a total loss, Dylan and I had another awesome hot date and as always, comedy kept saving me with every joke, notebook, and set.

I wanted to become a comedian so badly and reckoned this was part of a culture I had to endure in order to advance. But the severity of the pain had become a type of hiding, like leading a double life, when I lie all the time to my loved ones to protect them. Even worse: not acknowledging to myself just how much I hurt. One time I had a particularly successful set, then concluded with a heartily, "Don't forget, if feel charitable, fuck a gimpy," which had the audience roaring. Because earlier I'd said, "Ground rules: I don't fuck you—the able-bodied—out of pity, and neither do I want to get pity fucked!"

As I left the stage and went back to my table, the host hollered at the audience, "Don't say 'fuck a gimpy' Kaatje, because that's an S&M word. You guys know what I'm talking about." I looked over my shoulder, for once in my life finding words quickly, "Oh, okay, how about, fuck a cripple?!"

The audience laughed even harder. It was impossible to do an open mic without hosts trying to put me down. Although my riffing had improved, and my sets were getting better, it still felt like one long, relentless exercise in exile.

* * *

From the moment I started performing comedy, I believed that, if my comedy improved, and the audience liked me, one day I would be accepted. There was so much I had to conquer; my Dutch accent, worsening disability, insecurity, struggles with wheelchairs, mobility, getting to and from a venue, grief. All my genuine efforts, being naturally gregarious, and kind in my enthusiasm for the local comedy scene, even hosting the first Annual Comedy Awards was all for naught.

Being ostracized by the community—whether "deserved" by lying down in the wrong place, discrimination, competition, the good ol' boy network, personal dislike, or that my jokes were a little too close to home—was brutal. The word ostracization comes from the Greek word *ostrakon* 'to banish an unpopular or too powerful citizen from a city for 5-10 years, by popular vote. Sadly, in the spring of 2017, it dawned on me that I'd been unfriended by most of the Albuquerque comedy community. Not everyone; a few comedians approached me, said it was bullshit and advised me to keep going.

But no one stood up for me in public, or on-line, and so, even the few people who used to say hello and give me a hug, no longer did. Some no longer even made eye contact. One comedian visibly recoiled and turned his back to me, after I touched his forearm to say goodbye. Later on, it was confirmed that he was told to cease all contact with me. Remember those rhesus monkeys with a faux metal mother, who went unhugged, starved for affection and were dying from a lack of love?

Oh man that was sad! In his book *This is Not Fame* Doug Stanhope recommends not talking smack about another comics' performance, to avoid saying things like "S/he wasn't funny," since humor is so personal. An audience may love the comic that you despise, and vice versa. So, I agree with Doug. In theory.

Because this is what I never understood about local comedy: Why were promoters and comics, who'd harshly judged me and my physical situation, fine with featuring ableist, racist, homophobic sounding comics? "I dated this chick in a wheelchair once…she wasn't feeling it. Good thing she couldn't run away…she tried! I dated this Indian woman…she was an real Indian giver, she gave me an Indian burn down (points at his crotch, indicating *STD - K.G.*)."

After surviving that set, as an audience member, still supporting local comedy, I came out of the bathroom and rolled towards the headliner who was approached by Dylan. That was weird, Dylan usually doesn't initiate conversations. I enthusiastically joined the awkward duo, and very strongly shook/squeezed the comics' hand and said: "My set has a lot of jokes about disabilities too! Oh, you've met my boyfriend, nice." The now even more profusely sweating comic appeared aghast and exclaimed: "I don't believe this, you're together? An Indian and a woman in a wheelchair, you're dating? Fuck me!" Then he blabbered: "I was just telling your boyfriend that I joke about everyone, like fat people too, look at my gut."

Later on, I totally ripped *him* off, because this became one of my best jokes, about my wham-bam-thank-you-man: "So this hot guy was spanking me. He was really into it, kept spanking until I got so bored, turned around and said, 'You know what?…I'm not feeling it….Besides, if you wanna do some daddy shit you should probably flip me over and punch me in the face!" The one-nighter was a piece of shit. Probably angry all the time, because his botched circumcision had left him with a penis the size of a shrimp. And not one of those jumbo shrimps either.

(Which is no excuse, there's serious reasons why someone's sexual organs deviate from the norm, whether from birth or trauma—plenty vets have gotten their genitals blown off. Disease, illness and the side effects of medications cause impotence and low libido too. Hey, someone ought to write a one-woman comedy show about this, and other, stuff!)

* * *

Journalist Michael Kelly, killed in Iraq in 2003, once remarked that big evils, like Satan, or conspiracies, do not exist. I'm paraphrasing, but he said something like: "Real evil is the daily, small things people do to each other." People are clueless about the impact of their actions and words. No matter how minute the acts, they can have a permanent, severe consequence in the life of another. Just imagine how much better the world would be if we could realize the ripple effect our interactions have. Then, act accordingly, like, be a human with a heart.

I kept wondering why I wasn't accepted, particularly since the lifeline from my hospital bed to the outside world was determined mostly by comedy. Come to think of it, the questions ought to be: Why wasn't I accepted in any clique, ever? Would it be my fate to always feel disconnected from humanity?

Some part of me said, *Oh, but I must like it this way. There must be something that appeals to me; otherwise my life wouldn't have worked out differently.* I'd console myself by saying: *This road is harder but more interesting.* In this case, it meant developing my comedy, alone, and through perseverance. No high fives for me after a set, but no concessions either.

This path is not for everyone; but for an outsider, it's worth embracing. *Find your strength, build on it, find your weakness, learn from it. Accept yourself the way you are.* Mandeep's scribbled notes reminded me that I had to share this message with others, who faced similar challenges. If people are incapable of compassion, those who are outcasts must draw strength from inside, rather than from external affirmation. Lest not forget that bullying has an evolutionary function: rallying against a common foe—an outsider— increases cohesion.

I wondered if I just did not fit the mold. Too old and too disabled to belong, no matter how liberal the comedy community claims to be. But it's 2017. Where are all the gay, older, or disabled voices, locally and nationally? I know I'm not alone; rumors abound of other local comedians who have been driven out of the scene, for nothing more than personal dislike. On the other hand, when I googled *comedy cliques*, the advice was quite simple: "Are you chill, bro?" Meaning, to hang out with. Nope. I am not chill. Although this joke of mine rings true too: "I don't burn my bridges, I napalm the fuck out of 'm!"

I do have an easy smile, and uncontrollable urge to suck the bone marrow out of life. For most of my life, I've maintained happy-go-lucky ways that were, at times, a pretense, whereas other times, my affable ways were sincere. Nonetheless, it is also true that I'm a somewhat difficult woman who wants the truth more than group cohesion. Despite feeling lonely much of my life, I've always sensed that the price of admission into any group would be too high.

For all I know I did not give the hosts and comedians enough credit, or asked for too many favors, like going early. They've worked hard, for a long time, and Albuquerque is a tough town to make a living as a comedian. When I started out, I was gullible and impressionable, just wanted to make the audience laugh and forget about their sorrows for a few minutes—and get laid. About a year into working my ass of in the comedy scene, I was told: "You must understand, Kaatje, we're all working towards becoming professionals, so keep that in mind. This is no joke to us." No shit!

Then again, that snarky comment betrayed something ugly underneath. *How dare he assume that I, too, am not working to becoming a professional?* It was as if, by virtue of being severely disabled, I was never seen as a viable professional in my newfound vocation.

A comedy buddy once remarked that any comedy scene is mostly ableist, and a boy's clique. He said some hosts professed they hated me and my comedy. Whoa, I may not be the best or funniest comic out there, but that seemed a tad harsh, besides, audiences seemed to really like my sets. One fact remains, despite lifelong social and academic insecurities I've always been earnest, and too eager. Which surely may rub some people the wrong way.

I'd ask professors hard questions or showed them where they were wrong, when their own textbook showed the right answer. Not to put them on the spot, but to clear up contradictions, or improve the curriculum—although the latter I did behind closed doors. I meant no harm by any of it, but I'm slowly realizing my behavior may not have been neurotypical. Even if I'm not everyone's cup of tea, I did know this: I'm not a douchebag.

* * *

A lot of discourse stemmed from being, literally, in the wrong place, or environment and perhaps, not knowing when to shut up. Questions and discussions were welcomed by my professors at New Mexico Tech, not that I needed to do so often, because they're smart to begin with. But the world at large, is not my beloved Alma Mater. Sometimes I chose to leave employment, when it might have been more effective to speak up and defend myself. However, because society teaches it is best to only look as far as the disability, or to look away from the disabled individual, it is difficult to exert myself in ways that are expected in the larger culture.

The stigma attached to being disabled is often too much to bear. A good example is when I was working part-time at a large, Federal health care clinic as a Physician Assistant, prior to working in the nursing home with the long, carpeted hallways. My physical condition was deteriorating, and I hadn't yet received my adhesive arachnoiditis diagnosis. So, I was keen to make improvements, grow as a professional, and find ways to navigate more easily in the workplace.

Mobility, obviously, has been a longstanding issue. At this clinic, ordering physicians and PA-Cs went to the nurse's station to request tests or give further instruction. I asked the manager if I could text 'urinalysis needed in room 8' instead of making my way from the exam room to the nurses' station. I was limping with a walker or cane, rather than using my wheelchair at the time, because, invariably, the chair would worsen my sacral torment. It was an impossible situation. I liked my job there because I learned a lot from the providers, and patients appreciated me. I provided in-depth yet efficient care, and most importantly, patients felt understood.

When I suggested text messages, for speed and to save me the physical burden, the nurses, gang-like, refused. They claimed that using their personal phones at work would increase their monthly bills. *Huh. They use their personal phones to check Pinterest and Facebook all day long, yet, they're unwilling to use their personal phones for work-related business during their shifts?* In response, I came up with another solution: I purchased a Tracfone for $8 per month that I left at the nurse's station so I could text from my personal phone to the Tracfone, thus saving them any expense.

The nurses then argued, "We don't want to use your phone, what if it gets lost? Maybe you should use an electric scooter to get around, instead." The manager, who seemed to be waiting out her time until she could comfortably retire, decided to take away my private office and move me to the noisy, uncomfortable nurses' station—so I had to limp from there to the exam rooms, then backtrack to the computer station. Had I been an able-bodied person or full-time employee, I doubt that identifying an inter-office problem and providing a solution would have resulted in a similar punishment. It seemed that as a disabled woman, albeit with advanced credentials, I'm not treated with the same level of courtesy as someone with comparable skills and education.

* * *

It eventually became more common across the nation for clinicians to communicate with their nurses and medical assistants via text messages. My idea had been years ahead of the norm, but rather than acknowledge I'm someone with good problem-solving skills, I was bullied out of the workplace. No one stood up for me, and as a part-time employee, the atmosphere toward me became unbearable. One of the more senior physicians confided that I was not the first health care provider who had been bullied by the same group of nurses; I was the fifth or sixth PA/Nurse Practitioner who'd resigned.

I don't know whether their treatment was due solely to my disability or whether I was caught up in yet another illustration of how the War on Women impacts female relationships. Stepping back from my emotions, can I blame the female manager for her (in)actions? An article in *The Atlantic* explained why some women end up bullying other women in the workplace. [90]

In a male-dominated culture, women know there are only so many spots available for advancement, just as in other traditionally, male-oriented subcultures—such as the comedy community. That female manager, with a long history inside the patriarchy, cannot be counted on to help someone like me. In a competitive male-dominated workplace, vulnerable female members of the pack are driven out, and I made for an easy target. My comedy joke about The War on Women: "Oh, it's real, there's a 'War on Women.' The worst thing is, them byatches don't roofie me when they fuck me over!"

Instead of leaving the comedy community, like I'd left that clinic, I stubbornly stayed. I was hooked on comedy and on-stage performance; those few minutes on stage helped me combat my affliction. It was the only time when I was able to push the agony of my body to the back of my mind. In addition, it gave me a purpose for living, spending what time I could filling up notebook after notebook—not just to craft jokes artfully, but to connect my heart to an audience.

* * *

Prince gave so much of himself to his audience; he was one of the hardest working musicians who ever lived. Although I've never had a problem with opiate medication, and took fewer than prescribed, it's easy to see how my buddy Prince got himself into a bind. It seemed like he needed ever-increasing dosages of pain medication just to keep performing. It's feasible that Prince was a "fast" or "ultrafast" metabolizer of opioid medication.

In the end, it seemed he was unable to get through daily life without taking both prescribed and illegally obtained meds. It's a pity we lost touch because I surely would have told him about ketamine, which also helps with arthritic, bone and joint disease. [91] It baffles me that someone with that much money, and such a splendid reputation, did not have access to, or knew about, intravenous ketamine infusions.

Prince could afford the best private physicians, daily massages, a heated swimming pool in his own home, and a traveling physical therapist. Despite those resources, over the years his number of performances dwindled, which may have reflected the progression of his physical deterioration. Apparently, he suffered from severe hip and ankle pain and injuries, and from grave anxiety and stage fright—which I had not known when we met. Prince performed almost fifty times in 2007, but only played in Las Vegas, Nevada and at the O2 Arena in London, rather than touring in multiple locations.

There were no other concerts scheduled until 2010, during which he did a total of 18, mostly in his old stomping grounds of Europe and New York City. In 2011, Prince achieved another 60 concerts. That man pushed himself. And yet, he performed only eight shows in 2012, 30 in 2013, 13 in 2014, and none in 2015. In 2016, Prince toured again, but rather than a full-blown show, he sat at a piano for 12 magnetic, beautiful, intimate concerts. For those with the wisdom to see it, this style of entertaining signaled a warning about the severity of his tragic physical state.

* * *

Prince and I met in Paris at a fancy nightclub called L'Atmosphere when I was 17 and he was 28, at the height of his Purple Rain fame. Prince was thin, tiny and there was a frailty about him, in real life. I can only imagine that he had worn out his skeleton, performing for decades in high-heeled boots, jumping up and down for hours at a time. His was not the stocky, or naturally athletic, body that could handle those kinds of antics for decades.

"Will you come to Frankfurt on Sunday, on my private plane? I have a few more concerts, it'll be fun," he asked, at the end of the evening. We'd been chatting amicably since we met, just the two of us in a cordoned off VIP section without interruptions. L'Atmosphere was mostly an insider only nightclub, no wonder rock stars and famous movie stars such as Catherine Deneuve enjoyed it, without the *riffraff.*

"No, I have to work in a small village in the South of France," I replied. "A Coca-Cola commercial." "You know, I wished I could go to a small village, and be anonymous."

"But Prince, you could!"

"How?"

"It's easy," I said, eyeing his clothes, purple velvet pants, high heeled boots, his frilly white shirt and 80's frilly hair. From the moment I entered the 80's as a twelve-year-old I'd liked Joy Division and U2 but hated glam rock, pop music and 80's fashion. I knew his look was a trap.

"You put on a baseball cap, sunglasses, wear American blue jeans, a t-shirt and lose the bodyguards. Trust me, no one will recognize you. Come on, it'll be fun," I said enthusiastically, my long Dutch strawberry blond braids shaking.

I'd met his father too that evening, Roger Nelson, a seemingly kind man who was much more outgoing than Prince himself who spoke softly, almost shyly. Prince was always nice to me, and we had dinner every time he came to Paris for his European concerts. His old manager, Steve Fargnoli, would call me and arrange the restaurant, and the town car.

Prince's fame was such that we were stared at all throughout dining, with an occasional, daring fan approaching our table. As always, his bodyguards hovered around us. He signed a napkin for the older woman, who asked for one more, for each of her two grandkids. "No," Prince said. And that was all. No explanations, just his personal policy. And why not, what's the alternative, keep signing napkins for an hour, with some going to be sold? I didn't care for his fame, and yearned to eat unencumbered, in a small village town that somehow, we would never visit.

Although we lost touch over the years, I'm truly saddened for his agony. I'm equally troubled by how many others are needlessly burdened, by their body's torment but also by the stress of medical bills. Here's a disheartening thought: if Prince—not known for alcohol or drug addiction—didn't have adequate support to cope with his ailments despite his wealth, connections and medical opportunities, how are impoverished, chronic pain patients supposed to make it? Yet Prince's situation is also perfect example of exactly how difficult it is, to treat debilitating pain in an aging body.

Chronic pain sufferers often push themselves too hard. Perhaps most don't perform on stage, but there's a constant internal battle. How to regain lost mobility, to do what we were able to do *before* versus maintenance, to avoid losing even more functionality. As someone who obviously created more aches and dysfunction, instead of obtaining a power wheelchair or taking better care of my body throughout life, I truly regret my past decisions. Now that I'm older, I've realized that my lifelong pattern of overdoing it has brought me more misery than was ever necessary.

We're told by medical providers and therapists that movement and pushing the body beyond its limits is the path to healing; but often, it's the path to further disability. When you're in chronic agony it's easy to forget that physical pain is supposed to function as a warning signal. It's the body's way to tell the brain to stop doing whatever it is that worsens discomfort. I exercised relentlessly at times, but couldn't distinguish between my baseline agony, my chronic sports injuries such as trochanter and left shoulder bursitis, or my worsening neurological torment.

Don't get me wrong, exercise is critical, and despite how brutal it can be to get myself out of bed, I swim and stretch three times a week. It's important to remember that the right kind of exercise, limited in scope to what's appropriate, is key. However, forcing ourselves to do things that we physically weren't capable of, as Prince and I and millions of others have done, seldom brings a happy ending. Pacing myself was not in my vocabulary, or DNA. I was incapable of not overexerting myself and as a result, seemed to destroy my future.

9 THE QUEEN OF KETAMINE

*There are three things I was born with in this world, and there
are three things I will have until the day I die—hope,
determination, and song. - Miriam Makeba, South African singer
& UN goodwill ambassador*

Every infusion was different, but as soon as the ketamine reached the receptors in my brain and spinal cord, my body immediately felt relief, as if a burn was finally soothed by an internal ice pack. It was marvelous. Perhaps because I had done cadaver dissection, and I have an active imagination, but it felt as if the liquid calmed down my lumbosacral nerve plexus. I could feel every branch of those nerves rejoicing, my spinal cord stabilizing, trying to get to a pre-accident state.

By my ninth infusion, June of 2017, I was finally able to stay coherent throughout the treatment. I'd learned how to kick ketamine's ass; or rather, successfully fight the side effects. I was lucid enough to ask the affable, compassionate nurse what her real name was. "Mandy" just did not sound probable, and sure enough, her given name was Mandeep. Which means 'enlightened' or 'mind full of light.' I was a tad disappointed that she had never read *The God of Small Things* or *A Fine Balance*, two works of Indian literature equivalent to *War and Peace*, or Japan's epic works, *The Wind-Up Bird Chronicle* and *Mushashi*.

"Mandeep, *The God of Small Things* and *A Fine Balance* are simply must-reads," I said, feeling confident enough to call her by her real name. I felt a close association with the friendly nurse, a fellow hard-working immigrant who had made a success out of her life here in the States. I had once been successful too, even if I now felt like a failure, not being able to work the last few years. I was three hours into the infusion, my mind drifting around or into the Universe, my body finally content and experiencing less pain, with only negligible hallucinations and vivid dreams.

"Mandeep, they're the kind of books that will break your heart. Gently," I continued my sales pitch.

"I will consider but promise me you will see Hasan Minhaj's stand up special, he's an excellent Indian comedian on Netflix," she replied.

I solemnly swore, in my ketamine haze, with my limbs floppy and my mind even floppier, that I'd watch him. I was lying comfortably in the motorized La-Z-Boy, but then felt a metal plank pushing in my back and sacrum. This new chair was worse than the manual La-Z-Boy chair the clinic had provided before. I can never understand why clinics do not consult patients who are in chronic agony, before they buy furniture, 'cuz we're the folks who can offer the most definitive judgments! Then again, perhaps my personal history of sacral fractures and peculiar health problems meant the only way to be somewhat comfortable was lying down. Feasibly, there might not be a chair in the world that's suited to my needs.

My remark to Mandeep about those books by Indian authors was a bit of a white lie. Although the ketamine infusion was running at full speed, I was fully aware that those works conveyed so much truth about the human condition; their content will rip out one's heart, thoroughly. The kind of books that changes every reader. Mandeep turned off the drip, and when the infusion stopped, I remembered that Mandeep's mother had come over when her grandchildren were born. Give it up for mothers, all over the world! And, I recalled her recommendation to watch Hasan Minhaj's Netflix special. Even on ketamine, I always kept my promises.

* * *

Because of the seemingly miraculous pain-relieving effects, I'd learned how to tolerate and/or love the experience that ketamine afforded my mind. Although I now felt lucid, and more in control during the treatments, the dissociative anesthetic still took me for a mild spin. My neurons and consciousness would float up inside an elevator, far out into the Universe and beyond, a couple of galaxies over. But I would never experience a K-hole again, and for that, I was grateful. I did develop this irrational fear of sedating medications; if there were psychological side-effects, that to me was evidence the ketamine was working on healing my inflamed neurons. I didn't want benzodiazepines to compete with ketamine.

My intergalactic visions, no doubt, were rooted in latent memories of reading Arthur C. Clarke, Isaac Asimov, and Douglas Adams as a teen. These male authors' works were what I had access to at the time. Female sci-fi writers weren't translated to Dutch back then, and Tess Gerritsen hadn't yet published her brilliant books. And of course, I've loved most sci-fi movies and TV, except for *Star Wars* and *Star Trek*. I'm more of a Firefly, District 9 and Battlestar Galactica kinda woman.

I felt so at peace with the world, yet remained aware of my own suffering, especially these last few years. I've had a keen understanding of the tragedies associated with immigration, caste systems, war, and the poor's plight since I was a kid. There was something about this particular infusion that brought sharper focus on those lifelong concerns. But I needed a mental anchor, like that child's toy in *Deception*—rather than ask for medications that would diminish the physical, psychological and transformational aspects—so had asked Mandeep to play Miriam Makeba. I was raised on her music, long before I was born, as my dad was her biggest fan.

Perhaps this infusion was different because I finally reached a zero-pain level, and my mind felt freed from my decades-long—and constant—companion. Perhaps it was the nature of the drug itself. Perhaps it was another kind of breakthrough, one that I needed to propel my life forward, to push through to the next level. Whatever the cause(s), the experience was profound enough that I knew it was important to record. Mandeep was kind and took notes about what I deemed significant during the infusion, the deepest truths about my life and my observations about humanity.

After the infusion, she handed me a scrap of paper with the things I'd asked her to write down: "The Queen of Ketamine. Not born on American soil. Human comfort. Live life with a good heart." She'd added, "Hasan Minhaj!"

* * *

Those notes, and my observations during that infusion, were the seeds for this book. I had already attempted to write about my convoluted life years ago, chapters that culminated in a 324-page memoir. When it was finally done, in 2014 after five years of writing, I called it *Gravity*, but then, the Sandra Bullock movie came out. Fine. How about *Hard to Kill*? Well that turned out to be yet another bad Steven Seagal movie. Fuck you, Hollywood: you stole my youth, my health *and* my memoir titles!

I happily renamed it *The Night I Broke my Butt & Other True Stories*, but before I could revise in earnest, the physical torment hijacked my body and all hell broke loose in my life. Apparently, before any revision or a new memoir, I needed to become a comedian first. Ketamine was the finishing touch; with less pain, I was finally able to unleash the creativity that had been percolating for decades. It did feel as if, in my little life, my Universe, I really had become the Queen of Ketamine.

Feeling profoundly humbled and grateful to reconnect with my creativity sure beat the inkling I'd just spend half of my life feeling sorry for myself, suffering mightily from unrelenting and unimaginable physical hurt. I'd almost given up on living—on hope—altogether. That changed when I discovered ketamine as a treatment. For those who have severe neuralgia or neuropathy, in addition to many other diseases and disorders, the treatment shows promise. Sharing that message with others became my inspiration.

After my *Queen of Ketamine* breakthrough, and with a renewed sense of purpose, I was high as hell on life. When I say high, I mean feeling normal. When my physical suffering is controlled, endorphins can find their way through my brain again. I felt able to do things that, only a few years before, I believed would be forever beyond my grasp. I wanted to see my father for the last time, he was now careening into end-stage Alzheimer's. Finally, having long-lasting relief, I felt up to the journey and bought a plane ticket to the Netherlands.

* * *

Oh, Dad. I made it there in time, as he still recognized me, although he was no longer oriented to time and place. I finally saw the child he must have been before the abuse had hardened him. He couldn't stop talking about how beautiful the clouds and the leaves were, moving in the wind. My entire life, dad had refused to discuss his youth, even when asked about innocuous stuff, like growing up working class in Eindhoven, shivering in the winter with ice flowers on the window. I knew my dad was the first one in his family to go to college; he received an Engineering degree from Eindhoven Technical University.

Obviously, Alzheimer's had loosened his tongue, and for the first time, I heard my Dad talk about his youth, and his beloved father. Turns out my grandfather had surprised my dad by unexpectedly showing up during an engineering internship, in France. My father's thick tears cascaded down his cheeks when he recalled the fond memory of five, six decades ago. My grandfather had died from lung cancer when I was a few weeks old, I'd realized now that was one of the clouds hanging over my young life; my father's phenomenal grief.

"We saw a German plane go down, above the soccer fields, and he protected me. Pushed us in a ditch, and lied on top of me," he said all of a sudden, with a surprisingly clear voice. Then his bright blue eyes darkened and welled up with tears again, this time his face a mask of anger and bitterness.

"But my mother," he said, in an urgent, harsh whisper, "she was a mean woman. Made me look for her by the canal, in the dark, when she threatened to kill herself, again and again."

It had been important to fly home and say goodbye to my father. Perfect timing since it would be quiet; my brother, his Moroccan wife and their kids were vacationing in Morocco for seven weeks. I knew my well-meaning brother to stump all over my boundaries, so I enjoyed these peaceful mornings. For a month I had breakfast with dad while he "read" the newspaper twice and told the exact same stories about his childhood, teenage years and the friends he had as a young man, via an old photo album.

My mom had rented a chic electrical hospital bed, so much more elegant and functional than my American bed. Their home was L shaped and open, with a kitchen inside the shorter part of the "L", a dining area, a desk, and comfortable seating at the far end. The hospital bed was placed in the dining area, parallel to the large dining table facing the kitchen, and I had a perfect view on the kitchen as well as the rest of the home. My dad would drink his morning tea while occasionally looking up to observe the clouds through the long horizontal shaped window behind me.

Alzheimer's was made very real when one night, my dad ran around the living room naked, panicked because he terrified, saying he had been *bitten by a flea*. My mother had long been his sole caregiver, without even a day's respite. Even from the hospital bed, I managed to clean up, sell, donate most of their household as the house was going to be on the market soon. Mom and dad needed to move to a small apartment, but she was already a burned-out caregiver; dad wouldn't sleep more than an hour or two before waking her up with a perceived crisis.

* * *

Between the 18-hour flight to Europe, and the exacerbating circumstances I'd encountered during my visit, I undid all the progress I'd made between January and June of 2017. It wasn't from lack of trying. During my visit, my stellar primary care provider, Dr Moekti, had made another appointment for me with the Pain Team at the small, regional hospital. Dr Moekti intuitively grasped that due to aging, changing hormones, or from arthritis, my pain threshold had tipped, and I was losing the battle. He'd done his best to cheer me up, telling me I had a good heart and I was gonna be all right.

"No one is going to pay me a professional wage for having a good heart, Dr Moekti!" I'd replied, in tears. Despite the referral letter, the Ivory Tower had been even more fortified than the time I'd asked in 2015. A different physician then the one in 2015 had a similar attitude, he sneered at my request for ketamine treatment and said it was no longer offered.

"I don't understand. This morning, I saw your website state that in-patient ketamine infusions are on the menu. Especially for intractable pain," I said, begging him for relief. I told him I'd received ketamine infusions abroad and that they worked for me.

"I'm not convinced there is enough evidence to prove efficacy for neuropathic pain," Dr. Dipshit said with a contorted face, as if he couldn't get rid of a large turd.

"Besides," he continued with a smirk, "it's an unacceptable therapy if patients need infusions as many as two to three times a year."

I thought to myself, *Would cancer patients on chemo be told that five infusions are too much? If physicians explain that adhesive arachnoiditis pain is comparable to having Stage IV cancer-like pain—without the relief of death—why would they deny me infusions that could remedy my suffering? I bet if this 'klootzak' himself was in physical agony, he'd insist on a monthly maintenance infusion.*

The Dutch physician ended our visit by saying, "We will not discuss this any further. Our hospital no longer offers it, and there's nothing I can do for your neuropathy and complaints. Goodbye." I arrived home, in Albuquerque, destroyed. A storm had delayed flights, detouring me via Chicago and Denver, and a careless airport employee threw me out of my wheelchair, my poor body flying a few feet on the ramps' carpet, giving my hands rugburn.

My boyfriend awaited me on the other side, so I refused medical care. Despite a letter from my Primary Care Provider to provide accommodations, or an extra seat next to me, the United Airlines staff refused to help on three back-to-back flights, without any time to lie down at one of the airports. The inflight staff ignored me like the plague, when I could not hold back tears, crying loudly, trying to suppress screams from agony in the uncomfortable, hard, narrow seat. For 24 hours straight.

The only hope on the horizon was that my health insurance would approve a one-week stay at the Rio Grande Hospital for an extended, 24/7 ketamine infusion in their step-down ICU. Traveling all the way to Arizona for a series of four hour-long infusions was becoming too arduous for my ailing body. Furthermore, I wanted to try an inpatient treatment. And boy, by that time, did I need it.

* * *

I'm in the hospital on ketamine at 55 mg per hour, 24/7, and I keep reaching for my phone. By comparison, the outpatient clinic's ketamine dose added up to around 240 mg over three and a half hours. No music, I made that mistake once already during an outpatient treatment in the winter of 2017, when I'd listened to DJ Grammatik and Kruder & Dorfmeister. Turns out, electronic dance music and ketamine are incompatible, it gave me nightmares and felt as if the music permeated my bones. It was an awful experience, and since then, if I want sound at all, I stick to my beloved Miriam Makeba or relaxation music.

Inexplicably, the hospital team didn't recommend turning off my phone, so I ordered two sequin gowns from ASOS UK. I love Joan Rivers' comedy and her work ethic, and in my ketamine daze, I figured emulating her by wearing pink sequin gowns was a great homage. Thanks to the IV ketamine, I have very little eye-hand coordination, but I keep writing, as it feels good to have my fingers fly over my lightweight, Chromebook keyboard.

It's the least I can do right now. I was not convinced on the first night that this weeklong ketamine treatment was a good idea, but I am won over by the Pain Management's team and the hospital staff. I now somewhat favor inpatient, hospital-based ketamine, as for me, lying down in bed is much more preferable for me than even the most comfortable La-Z-Boy. The hospital-based IV ketamine treatment has added IV magnesium, which is another medication that works on the NMDA receptor and may have a synergistic effect by giving ketamine a boost.

Even on ketamine, I remain too sensitive to other people's emotions. Earlier today I had a great conversation with nurse Lucy, explaining how my physical anguish is a 7 today, as I reserve a 10 for slamming into the ground at 70 mph. Lucy had a hard time, at first, understanding how much agony I'm in. She made a remark that most people who are here for ketamine infusions are, "Hunched over and complain about their clothes hurting them." But I'm not here to complain about my affliction; I'm here to improve. Besides, the more I tell myself how miserable I am, the more miserable I will feel.

Plus, they bring me meals three times a day, and I have a private room and bathroom. Since I'd arrived at the hospital hungry, unable to take care of myself, this was a win-win situation. How isn't this one of the happiest weeks of my post-accident life?! Lucy returned and then became preoccupied when she had to ask another nurse about why they couldn't read the blood pressure values on the monitor from the day shift. They putzed around with the blood pressure monitor and disclosed that I had spiked to 201/92.

The previously kind Lucy made no eye contact and ignored me—no one even asked how I was feeling or if I had a headache given that high blood pressure. Secretly, I was like, *Please let me stroke out*, but on the other hand, I was finally enjoying a lot less suffering, and just thought, *Oh, so there is life at the end of the tunnel. Maybe I would like to keep on living, after all.* I make a mental note to bring in my own blood pressure monitor, because frequently the cuff is put on too loose or too tight, or after a strenuous bathroom visit.

* * *

So often it feels like I am writing in a void. However, my quiet morning is interrupted by a lot of things: email, texting, and strengthening the bonds of family and friendship. And at the end of your life, or during a crisis or a hospital stay, trust me, those bonds are much needed. It doesn't matter how many friends you have on Facebook, if you have three people who will visit you in the hospital, and one of them is your younger, risk averse and introverted boyfriend, another an old friend from PA school, and the third is an acquaintance who suffers chronic neuropathy too, that is enough.

And if, in your deepest, darkest hour, you have two friends you can call, one of them your Mom, and another your best friend since your teens, you have a rich life—thanks to the ketamine I temporarily forgot how lonely I often feel in my hospital bed at home! Suddenly, I feel tired for trying so hard to fit into other people's lives. I have a seven-lead EKG on my chest, and with the infusion going and a nasal cannula for supplemental oxygen sticking out of my nose, it's getting harder to write.

But I wanted to recall in the future, how precious this life is. How few seconds we have, and to remember how Mandeep made me aware of the vital importance of human comfort, through our chats about her kids. It does not matter how many Twitter followers one has, and it is a waste of precious, limited time wondering how many real friends a Kardashian has. (I do want to know, never having watched their reality series, although they seem happy in pictures.)

A nice Nigerian Tech brought my lunch, a delicious curry with tofu, and we both agreed the kitchen needed to provide way more curries. The same day I had another fortunate encounter, with a cleaning lady who longed to return home to Mexico. "No bueno, los Estados Unidos." Lupe was a sweetheart and took time to chat, I enjoyed our little interactions. Perhaps the entire world ought to be on ketamine, at least once. A lesser known, but annoying side effect of ketamine is a feeling of grandiosity: for example, having delusions of importance and coming up with nifty plans for say, eradicating malaria. (Malaria is relatively easy to eradicate, via DDT impregnated mosquito nests and handheld DDT sprayers. With millions killed since well-meaning people thought DDT was *no bueno*, thank goodness DDT's making a comeback.)

That's why I really admired Dr Rogelj's patience with me. Luckily grandiosity would plague my mind only during the first weeklong treatment —usually I just feel overjoyed, my mind not encumbered by smarting. Dr Rogelj is the head of the Pain Management team, and yet he visited daily to document progress during my first ever inpatient treatment. Today though he looked a little annoyed, as I set forth the UN resolutions that would broker forever peace between Palestine and Israel.

Interestingly, Dr Rogelj and I had crossed paths when he was a resident in Pain Medicine and Anesthesiology in 2006. After an epidural steroidal injection by his preceptor, he diagnosed me with hypertension. Sometimes it was a little hard to understand him, he'd never lost his Slovenian accent.

"Me, hypertension?" I'd said incredulously. "I just had an invasive procedure. I'm in my thirties and in *perfect* health, other than the sacral nerve damage, the 70-mph landing, the inability to sit and having lost 2 inches of spinal height." Or something to that effect.

Recall that at the time in Physician Assistant school fulltime; the prolonged sitting in lectures caused so much physical pain, I endured multiple epidural steroidal injections at the lumbosacral level, and steroidal shots for my perpetually inflamed left *trochanter* aka hip bone from an altered gait. At home, I studied in a brown, secondhand La-Z-Boy, in the classroom I had a cushiony chair and in the cadaver lab a thick, padded garage stool in a saddle shape from Costco. I was beyond exhausted, from coming up with solutions to fit in an able-bodied world.

"Are you sure, Dr Rogelj?" I said. *Like I need another medical diagnosis. No way. No fucking way.*

"Look," he replied, "people who do not have essential hypertension may see a change to 130, 140 over 80. But you just had a blood pressure of 165 over 95. That is not normal. Go see your primary care provider."

I'm not completely daft so went the next week and I've been on lisinopril, hypertensive medication ever since. If Dr. Rogelj hadn't been persistent and diligent, it may have been another few years till I got treated. Because hypertension is silent, there are no symptoms until a first cardiac event. Of course, severe pain doesn't help either and may increase someone's blood pressure.

* * *

"Dr Rogelj," I said on my last day as an inpatient, "why has the neuropathy changed in quality? It is almost a buzzing kind of ache, a few times a week."

"I don't know," he answered cheerily, now that I had quit yapping about Middle Eastern peace.

"What do you mean, buzzing sensation?"

"Well, you know how as a child you leaned against a farmer's fence? The kind with a low voltage, to keep the cows confined?"

He looked quizzically, and gruffly said, in his thick accent, "You and I probably had a very, very different childhood."

I decided not to push my look and explain how the most daring of children would lick the wiring. Dr Rogelj said his goodbyes and, as is his custom, shook my hand strongly and kindly.

Strangely, during this hospitalization I've become more fearless in love and such matters, as it makes no sense worrying about whether I am young enough for my boyfriend. We'd never addressed the age difference, he's a Millennial and I'm a Gen-Xer. Dylan grew up on the Rez, in a mobile home, coincidentally in the same village where I did two internships as a Physician Assistant student. I happen to love small, dusty desert towns *and* mobile homes, so figured we had a lot in common.

An easier explanation is that I simply could not resist Dylan's artist way of thinking, his kindheartedness and his beautiful eyes. My father's close friend

King Sie had the same handsome eyes, as did my Dutch-Chines childhood dentist. As an immigrant, I've always been fond of other cultures and experiences, and from traveling all over the world learned there definitely is more that unites us than divides us. Our shared human history is heartbreaking, yet beautiful. And tough! As modern humans, can you imagine migrating across the Bering Strait, or making your way out of Africa, on foot?[92]

Interestingly, Native Canadians are known as First Nation, which makes it easier to grasp the concept that the North Americas were already populated, long before Europeans arrived. Genealogy is amazing stuff: technically, I am not even fully Homo Sapiens thanks to my 4% Neanderthal DNA. Although I'm proud of my heritage, I think it's the Neanderthal traits that have gotten me in trouble for most of my life! Apparently, I have 298 more Neanderthal variants than 83% of 23andMe customers, perhaps it's time to find my long-lost family.

Two days ago, my IV broke, and while I had to wait 20 minutes for someone to start a new one, some of the left leg and sacral pain returned, and it frightened me. Dylan had held my hand, saying just the right things. It seemed like no matter what, he loved me. The week had flown by, and I learned the hard way why everyone always complained of exhaustion after a hospitalization: the IV machines bleep, you get woken up for vital signs at all hours, and good sleep is hard to come by. On the other hand, sleep at home is impaired by gut-wrenching ache, so I didn't mind that much.

* * *

I'm back home, hours after the in-patient infusion, and now that I am no longer moaning from pain, I realize how ketamine has transformed my perceptions. Comedy, at first, was a defense mechanism against my bedridden, crippled life. Like all the defense mechanisms before, it seems like I tried to prop up my frail ego and combat my profound internal insecurities. And yet, I threw myself before a group of strangers and fellow comedians while hurting on levels well in excess of my physical agony. But comedy kept me going. I had a boyfriend who believed in me, and friends along the way, even if my social circle kept shrinking.

The physical torment that worsened from the comedy sets at the bars and other venues went unacknowledged, no one knew the price I paid for those few minutes of shining on stage. I was used to persevering, just as I had when the top of a mountain was another three hours away and engulfed in fog. It was a matter of putting one foot in front of the other. Our family slogan while hiking was *slow but steady*, although my personal moniker had been more in alignment with *fast and furious*. The future seemed hopeless, but I kept working on my stage material while I swam, or sat in the hot tub, being about as comfortable as I could be given the adhesive arachnoiditis. Nothing, and no one could stop me.

I had no plan in mind, except to keep writing comedy every day, no matter how bad my day was. At home in my hospital bed, imprisoned by my body, my mind thought of set lists, I rehearsed jokes, and I slowly started improving. As always, I wrote in my notebooks while lying on my right side, an icepack on my sacrum. I fought my fears of performing and struggled with feeling like an outcast. Even if I did my best set yet, no one gave me a high five. But the audience responded, and that was all that mattered.

There were no high fives for mountaineering, either, especially on solo hikes. I'd reach the top, and then the long trek down started, followed by another ascension, and I carried that attitude, and those experiences with me into my incapacitated, bedridden life. Although I had slowly been forced to get used to the lack of nature in my life, I missed the smell of the mountains.

It was so fresh and lovely up there, as if Earth tectonics had evolved only to produce that clean smell of rock and mist. Perhaps there was no end to the physical torment of my reality, but I kept going, mentally setting one foot in front of the other. My mountaineering memories lingered on, melancholically, while my olfactory system happily recalled the scent of the Tour du Mont Blanc trail at 2700 meters.

Occasionally, I would ask someone to record my gigs, but I never dared to look at the footage, I was too embarrassed. Not because of my disability, although that sometimes played into it. The thought of watching myself struggling with a mic cord or taking too long to get my power wheelchair elevated and positioned was almost too much to bear. Yet there was another, much deeper fear of watching myself which originated in early childhood. My dad obsessively photographed and documented our lives, every second, whether I wanted to or not. I was destined to exist in front of the camera, when I was sure my life could have had a greater purpose.

* * *

The lovely, talented woman who put me on this planet, while almost killing me with our shared umbilical cord wrapped around my little neck, was of no help either. I was born blue, and asphyxiated. I had pestered her throughout my life, asking why I was here and why it seemed I was raised by wolves. I even had wolf shaped fangs, being born with only two instead of four upper teeth (incisors), the two cuspids (sharply pointed canines) next to them. Grrrrr.

"We tried, honey. We enrolled you in team activities, and group sports but it never worked. You usually didn't like the other kids, and the feeling was mutual," she said softly during a phone call.

"Why did you have children, Mom?" I'd asked, aged six or seven, lying on their thick, woven orange and brown 1970s bedspread.

"Your Dad and I love each other, and in those days, you started a family," she'd replied, exasperated, while she was folding laundry with her muscular arms and freckled hands. This wasn't the first time I'd cornered her.

"You didn't think about it much beforehand, did you?"

"We're very happy to have you. Besides, I lost a child when I was pregnant, before you."

"Whoa Mom, too much information."

"Sweetie, we were going to name you Saskia, after the 14-year-old daughter of close friends, but she died a week before you were born, so we named you Kaatje," she added.

"How do people die, mom, like this?" I asked, confused, lying on their bed with my arms now positioned in a 90-degree angle and my legs crossed at the ankle, just like the crucifixes sprinkled across the Catholic countryside.

"Saskia died while riding a bike, sweetie. People die in all sorts of ways. We don't believe in Jesus, that figure you've seen hanging on a cross. Some folks are what we call 'religious,' and they have a religion called Christianity. Christ is another name for Jesus, but your Dad and I are sure religion is all hearsay and hysteria."

Suffice it to say that I have never found a satisfying answer to why I existed, and yet, comedy was the first outlet that made me feel as if a better life, or a better me, was possible. It became my faith. When I started performing, aside from struggling with the mic cord, I was only vaguely aware of being disabled, or female, or an older comedian. To me, my external circumstances didn't seem to matter much, for my inner battles were more encompassing.

A friend of mine, comedian Kris Shaw, once said that you don't choose comedy, comedy chooses you. Kris added, "She's a harsh mistress." And She is. I feel beyond blessed comedy choose me on that day of my diagnosis. It was as if a fountain inside of me opened. There was no stopping the ideas, the observations, the punchlines, and the elaborate jokes. Comedy was also more than an outlet for my creative personality. Comedy was the engine that would define my destiny.

Those early childhood experiences carried over to how I dealt with my injuries. Never once did I lament, after my skydiving accident, *Why me?* Instead, I always thought, *Why not me?* Thousands of people are injured every year, with complete or incomplete spinal cord injuries. Because I'm pragmatic, I'd say to myself, *Well, I can't complain now. I shouldn't have jumped that night.* But I did ruminate, and for years, I was consumed by profound guilt over my accident, until I finally sought help from a counselor at New Mexico Tech. I felt that I'd done something so stupid, an act so devoid of reasoning, I would never forgive myself for that skydive.

* * *

Yet I stumbled upon some type of healing; having done real, stand-up comedy mere weeks after my adhesive arachnoiditis diagnosis in 2015. I wasn't half as proud of my former accomplishments, such as becoming a Physician Assistant, because truthfully, I was ashamed that I had to skip a semester, and left two PA schools to recover from the arduous academic adventures, bullying by lecturers and/or lack of disability help. Though I profoundly regretted my ill-fated decisions, like arguing with professors— even if I was usually right.

I was ashamed it took me eleven years to finally obtain my Master's in physician assistant studies, from the time I started at Oakland Community College. My cheeks and chest burn profusely, contemplating why I did not prioritize my health and, in the process, perhaps inadvertently, sacrificed my marriage. Although, Jeremy and I got super hooked on *Battlestar Galactica* and oh boy, was Season Three depressing, or what? They're stuck on a muddy rock, where it rained all the time, and to this day, I quip, "BSG, Season Three is what really fucked my marriage."

And yet, throughout hospitalizations and setbacks, comedy kept me tethered to this life. Comedy got a hold of my soul, and as I worked through joke after joke, and filled one notebook after another, I grew serious cojones. I've always been obdurate, but experienced real fortitude, to get me through life, and the courage to tell the truth. Sadly, I'm not sure how much longer I'll be able to do live stage performance.

I've learned that living with intractable pain is a constant lesson in adaptation. Being able to adapt is the secret; I'm getting ready to accept life with chronic anguish that will never end. But, I'm a trooper. I can write from my bed, and I have the internet, and if I can't go to the audience in person, maybe I can use YouTube. I've realized that while making people laugh is equivalent to an adrenaline high, perhaps it is not the comedy life itself that I'm after. It's the ability to connect with people, to connect my heart to the good in humanity.

* * *

I've learned how to be a tad kinder to my body. The first week after the hospitalization I even made a salad, bought by a kind friend. I took the salad, the gorgonzola crumbles, and the dressing from the fridge. There was a pleasant absence of discomfort in my arms—no allodynia from the cold air escaping from the fridge, hurting me. I sat on my upholstered barstool with a cushion, added tuna and peanuts from the generic Shurfine brand by John Brooks. I fucking love generic.

I finished the salad—iceberg, not my favorite—but my friend bought whatever was cheapest, and I remain amazed at this bountiful life, with affordable products in supermarkets. I carried the 'meal salad' (a Dutch expression; a large salad with nourishing ingredients, eaten as a complete meal) and climbed in bed, exhausted from the food prep, my lower legs and sacrum throbbing. I knew it was time for a huge rest, as in, being in bed the rest of the evening.

Before the meal prep, I'd spent an hour writing at my table, on top of a light-yellow tablecloth with embroidered flowers made seven decades ago by my maternal grandmother. I'd written cards and organized one binder—no small feat—as I had not sat at a table comfortably for years. Usually I can't write to friends and family, an activity I've enjoyed my entire life. I would pass out from worse physical suffering, and fatigue, after sitting upright, doing the smallest of tasks, and I spent many an evening crying from frustration.

Prior to my weeklong ketamine infusion at Rio Grande Hospital, once again I'd subsisted on ice cream, potato chips and/or gummi worms, stuff that requires no preparation and is easy to eat while lying down in bed. My visitor that same evening, a depressed friend who unfortunately also suffers from severe social anxiety, was a bit mad at me for suggesting she try a ketamine infusion.

"It's just another crappy day in my crappy life," she said, "You're still in bed, so I can't see how ketamine did you any good." *Ha! Ketamine and its pain reduction have saved my life.* I just wrote two pages, and although my sacrum hurts, it is nothing like before. Even if I'm mostly housebound, I went from being completely bedridden and wanting to die, to having a nice evening at home.

That is no minor miracle. It is as if my body and brain soaked up the ketamine, and it's exactly what I needed. And, as The Queen of Ketamine, I remained fairly lucid for a full weeklong treatment, save an outburst of grandiosity. My entire body, from T4 all the way to my toes, feels better. More normal. Although it's hurting, my left leg no longer feels like it's in a meat grinder, and the sensation of someone pounding a hammer on my sacrum is far less intense. My loyal companion, the perpetual torment, is a miraculous two out of ten. This is heavenly.

10 BACK INTO THE ABYSS

Success is not final, failure is not fatal. It is the courage to continue that counts. - Winston Churchill, British Prime Minister and writer

Four weeks out of the hospital and my daily life did not look so rosy anymore. The week after I was discharged, I overdid it, again. I will always remain my own worst enemy, but Rio Grande Hospital carried some of the responsibility. After the seven-day infusion, I was instructed to see my Primary Care Provider. Being a diligent patient, I followed their advice.

Since I'd sold my minivan, there weren't many transportation options available, especially since I had very few friends left, and I hadn't made any new ones since becoming bedridden 20/24 hours a day. I'd once made the 45-minute trip by public bus in my power wheelchair, but it took an entire day, and left me in much more physical agony. I do have a Sunvan pass for the disabled, but the struts on their vans are too stiff, worse than a public bus.

I decided to rent a car as all other options were harmful to my spine and exacerbated my pain. While I had the car with a three-day weekend special, it felt as if I had just been released from jail. Less restrained by physical agony, and feeling invincible for the first time in years, I went to Target on a Sunday morning, with my manual wheelchair. Of course, the shopping trip triggered an acute flareup. *You'd think I'd finally learned my lesson, but oh no.* I had no reserves left to make it to Meadowlark, a 30-minute drive on Monday. Complicating matters was my acute lack of home health caregivers.

Home health care assists with general housekeeping, such as bringing groceries, loading and unloading the dishwasher, laundry, and vacuuming, among other housekeeping tasks. These activities are simple matters for the able-bodied, but they are monumental feats for me. Without these services, my living space is dirty and cluttered, and every time I do any one of these housekeeping chores, it takes a breathtaking toll on my body. After the Lovelace Rehabilitation in 2015 I was allocated 20 hours a week, later decreased to 12 upon my request, when I moved downtown to a small studio.

Equally troubling; after the hospital discharge, Dr. Sol, the fantastic, smart hospital pharmacist/clinician, accidentally prescribed the wrong size opioid—

very tiny oxycodone 5 mg instead of the large, oxycodone 5 mg/acetaminophen 325 mg tablets. The pills prescribed were so small they could not be split in half, even with a pill cutter. I strive to keep my dosages low, so I normally only take half of a 5 mg tablet.

I took the prescription to my wonderful neighborhood pharmacy, Albuquerque City Drug, but they only had enough pills to fill half of the script. I thought one phone call to the hospital pharmacy would rectify the mistake—or mine, perhaps I did not clarify I needed acetaminophen with the oxycodone, which makes for a much larger, easy to break tablet. So, like a dummy, I told Albuquerque City Drug that I did not want the rest of that prescription, another 45 tablets. Three weeks and nine phone calls later, I don't have the correct medication and I am running really low on opioid medication.

* * *

As I am typing this, my left leg and sacral affliction have returned, not up to an 8 or a 9, but in the 6-7 range. I maintain that an 8 or a 9 is not compatible with life, but 7 is not much better, as that renders me completely bedridden. It is almost worse to have a 7 day than it was before I discovered ketamine. I was at a 2 when I was in the hospital. Now that I have recent memories of being nearly torture-free, the torment creeping back up almost seems to hurt more than it did before the weeklong infusion.

After all these years, *pacing* my activities remains hard. Because my pain and energy level had improved for a few days, against my better judgment, I'd participated in an Occupational Therapy photo shoot at the University of New Mexico; then attended the subsequent photography exhibit awhile later, taking a public bus with my power wheelchair. It took weeks to recover from each event. I'm starting to suspect however that I do things to avoid the isolation, and the feelings of overwhelming despair from not participating in life, and not contributing to society.

I cannot accept my frailty. I must resign myself to a life lived in bed, and perhaps, five minutes of comedy every week or two. I had been pushing myself to do two or three sets a week, but now I've gotten to the point where I can only make it out every so often. I'm growing even more isolated, more frustrated with the noise issues in my building, and now, I'm dealing with a whole new hurricane: the sudden, forced change from Medicaid to Medicare. It chokes and overwhelms me.

It turns out that my home health care is no longer reimbursed by Medicare, unless I'm on a ventilator – and I don't have the financial resources to spend $500 a month on care. I will lose the caregiving support system that took me months, years to build. Once again, I will be at the mercy of my very few friends to help me with my housework, obtain groceries, and maintain some semblance of independent living. I've made over twenty phone calls to the agency, and there is no one who can tell me how to avoid this lapse in my care. I ask Medicare, Medicare sends me to Medicaid. I ask Medicaid, they send me back to Medicare.

Meanwhile, my pain medication problem has yet to be resolved. Every time I call the hospital about the prescription mistake, their robot voice tells me: "We're experiencing a high call volume, call back later," and hangs up on me. I called Medicare again today, and the system said, "Too many agents are too busy, remember the busiest times to call are early in the month and early in the week," and then Medicare hung up on me too!

Not only are there new and devastating changes to my Medicare coverage, but they are so understaffed they cannot pick up the phone. Rather than hire and train more people to handle the calls, the government created specialized help centers for patients to provide in-depth counseling to cope with the psychological fallout of having to navigate the system. That's right, you must call a government-funded counseling center, called SHIPs. Their website proclaims:

The State Health Insurance Assistance Programs (SHIPs) provide free, in depth, one-on-one insurance counseling and assistance to Medicare beneficiaries, their families, friends, and caregivers. SHIPs operate in all 50 states, the District of Columbia, Guam, Puerto Rico, and the U.S. Virgin Islands, and are grant-funded projects of the federal U.S. Department of Health and Human Services (HHS), U.S. Administration for Community Living.

Clearly, this is a SHIP without a captain. Does the Constitution even matter? Because I am sure the Founding Fathers could not have imagined a government program so complicated, and layered with managers, that a nationalized insurance program cannot be understood by the people who work there. Is this why Medicare fraud is so easy? The federal workforce is not to be blamed either; America's workers in general do not seem the tough, make-do crowd of years ago. I mean, my local MVD closes when there's three or four snowflakes. Aside from SHIP, an organization named Medicare Rights has a mission statement that reads:

> *The Medicare Rights Center is a national, nonprofit consumer service organization that works to ensure access to affordable health care for older adults and people with disabilities through counseling and advocacy, educational programs and public policy initiatives. Since 1989, we've been helping people with Medicare understand their rights and benefits, navigate the Medicare system and secure the quality health care they deserve. We're the largest and most reliable independent source of Medicare information and assistance in the United States.*

Their slogan is "Getting Medicare Right." How pathetic: Medicare health insurance is so dense and bureaucratic it needs yet another *donation-based* organization to help patients—like me—navigate? Even with two bachelor's and a master's, I couldn't figure it out! There is nowhere to go with my anger and rage about this sheer volume of incompetence. This is much, much worse than the movie *Brazil* by Terry Gilliam. This is worse than even the two most well-known dystopian novels, *1984* and *Brave New World*, ever envisioned. It is a world made purely for people with healthy bodies and people who are able to work. Anyone outside the norm drops off a steep, deep cliff.

* * *

I've lost my BCBSM Medicaid and will be forced on Medicare in less than a month—once you apply for disability and are approved, you automatically qualify for Medicaid. This is what no one tells you beforehand: if you've been on disability for two years, you will be switched to Medicare. Because the system fails to provide help or guidance about this lapse in coverage, I have caregiving only until the end of the month.

A few weeks later, I offered to pay Jenny, my caregiver, out of pocket a couple of times. Just when I needed help the most, she texted she could not work because of a sore throat. She'd had a negative Strep test yet was anxious she'd make me ill. So, I told her I'd run the risk if she washed her hands; we all get viral infections six to eight times a year, which manifests as a sore throat and the sniffles for a few days, and I wasn't particularly worried.

But she never showed up for work. Another caregiver, who had worked with me for months, once again pushed the wrong buttons on the dishwasher. I swear, monkeys are easier to train than some caregivers. Instead of feeling sad or processing the grief over my worsening health—compounded on by lack of reliable caregivers—I'd spend the next few weeks in my hospital bed obsessing over science and agriculture. I'd resorted to ice cream, LAY'S® Limón potato chips and gummi worms for breakfast, lunch, and dinner, without a home health care aid doing groceries.

The sad thing is Walmart no longer sells *regular* salad in a box. You have to buy organic, which is more expensive. That's not democracy, that's a vocal few dictating US grocers to stop selling regular salad. I would be fine with a choice, one box organic, the other regular, or inorganic—at 75 cents, or a dollar cheaper. But we don't have that choice. And it affects the poorest population, who is better served adding much more fruits and vegetables, than scaring us that pesticides are killing us. Luckily, science backs me up.

And unless you live in Flint, tap water should be your go-to instead of buying one-time use plastic bottles, your teeth will thank you too—fluoride is your friend.[93] I have a serious addiction to *Popular Science, Popular Mechanics, Scientific American, Discover* and *New Scientist*. The latter only accidental, because as a Gen X-er, I had yet to figure out how to disable *New Scientist*'s notifications on my smart phone screen.

These little messages drive our dopamine levels up, and incentive people to read "Mass of a white dwarf star directly measured for the first time," or "What it's like to take psychedelics in small doses at breakfast," or "Artisan sourdough? You may as well eat mass-produced white bread."[94] *Oh, that third one is brilliant.*

I've never understood the now-trendy American obsession with tap water, GMO-free products, gluten sensitivities, and miniscule traces of pesticides. Few people realize that Norman Borlaug's *Green Revolution* allowed mass farming techniques to feed people, even in countries where humanity's greatest threat was famine. When put into practice, his ideas were responsible for the success of mankind and its expansion. Oh, overpopulation? I'm not worried. We're almost at peak human.

* * *

My daily life is about survival, as an organism, so forgive me for not giving a fuck about organic. If you have the physical and mental energy to worry about organics, count your blessings. People who suffer *food insecurity*, like me, seem to lack the ability to worry about politics, glyphosates, and Earth. (Food insecurity is the state of being without reliable access to a sufficient quantity of affordable, nutritious food.) Yet I am also proud, and overjoyed, with so many positive changes for the environment, even in my lifetime, such as the switch from lead in gasoline, the awareness of nicotine and lung cancer. And occasionally, I do worry.

About how dangerous coal mining is, how rare earth minerals like those used in solar panels and electronics are not recyclable, and why, if we are serious about energy, we don't invest in fourth generation nuclear reactors. France has 75% nuclear energy, and let's face it, solar and wind energy has a storage problem. What worries me most is the lack of clean drinking water and indoor sanitation for developing countries, and the fact that *3.8 million people* a year die from cooking indoors on wood fire, biomass and kerosene stoves, mostly woman and children.[95]

I also worry about prostitutes being underpaid, which ironically is an excellent joke, "Back in the 80's the Saudis would offer 'models' $3500 a night. Sure, I had friends who'd get fucked like a donkey by a coked-up Saudi prince, but hey those were the glory days. Last I heard $20 buck gets you a bum fuck in a Las Vegas alley, no lube. Aren't *you* guys worried about the deflation of whores?"

The irony is that all of that joke is true, and there are many reasons why sex workers are underpaid and why it's become *less* safe since Backpage was seized, and Craigslist stopped their personal ads. "And yes, I did choose the wrong side of that profession, but I was like, 'Oh, I have ethics. I got paid $90 a day to pose for Elle!' But seriously, I see some of you thinking; wow, I would like to get fucked like a donkey for $3500 a night."

Nah, my own fears and anxieties circle around keeping myself alive – literally – and feeling as though I am nothing but a sad bag of bones, muscles and brain. All of it, all of me, confined to a hospital bed in my studio, the lumbosacral adhesive arachnoiditis hijacking and wrecking my already meager existence. I wish I could be more like one of my favorite musicians, Curtis Mayfield. After his 1993 accident in Brooklyn left him with quadriplegia, he remarked, "This is just another experience."

When I last saw John Geven and Nicole van der Maazen, I'd asked, "How do you cope with caregivers, John? And the lack of independence?" to which he answered, with a slight shrug, "What choice do I have, really?" Eerily prescient, a good six months before I needed daily caregiving myself. When we were younger, after Hoensbroek I vaguely recalled he told a caregiver, "Not my problem, you wanted kids!" if his caregiver was going on and on about her baby crying through the night. But maybe I misremembered, or he'd mellowed throughout the years, running his successful photography studio, while being married and caring for his niece and nephew. Either answer worked for me.

* * *

Manual Therapy had helped the last few months, physically and mentally, but I finally had to acknowledge my therapist asked intrusive questions like, "Can you have orgasms?" Manual Therapy is like haptonomy—a specific Dutch massage/Physical Therapy treatment—where trust between a provider and a patient helps the body and mind heal. It is very effective, but since my weeklong ketamine treatment I changed, and realized the appropriate boundaries between therapist and client are not intact.

Last time I saw him, Mr. Manual Therapist placed his hand on my sacrum's most tender spot, where the fractures and scar tissue have left the nerves with constant agony, right underneath the skin. I yelled out, tears in my eyes when he touched the area, twice in one session! Which cost $90 for 1.5 hours out of pocket. I must have pointed out that specific spot at least a half dozen times in six previous sessions.

Besides, I was in cahoots with city officials. The City of Albuquerque promised to get back to me within five business days and it has been fifteen. Then thirty days. I pay property taxes, and I need someone to call me back about an issue in my building. Hey local, state, and federal government, I'm still human, despite being disabled. I call them every day and it's exhausting.

Maybe that's just life, but often it seems as though people have determined that, because I'm not able-bodied, I don't have the same rights as others. *How do I get my hands on the keys to a better life*? We, the frailest of society, are the forgotten people, buried underneath layers and layers of bureaucratic incompetency, left to rot by those too selfish, or not compassionate enough, to realize that the vulnerable members of society are the ones who most need the help. And what *is* my suffering compared to that of a sore throat?

Feeling lonely, I reached out to a dear friend, who knows how isolated I am. She texted back, asking how the Occupational Therapy photo exhibit went, to which I'd invited her. I was too exhausted to reply in detail and texted, "I value your friendship but prefer seeing you face to face, even if it's once or twice a year. Come visit me, you're a few minutes away by car!" She replied, "You do your thing, I do mine, no harm, no foul." *Huh?* Never heard from her again.

I know my symptoms are worsening, even though I had the recent in-patient ketamine infusion. I also know I've overdone it in the last month, doing house chores by myself. Perhaps the adhesive arachnoiditis progresses to *arachnoiditis ossificans*, and with how bad I'm feeling, I'm a tad terrified, because I'm fucked if that happens. It's a slow, agonizing process that turns the lumbosacral nerves into calcifications. That's right: the nerves turn into bone deposits. It is rare, but after developing two rare pain syndromes and surviving a horrifying skydiving accident, I'm no longer optimistic that won't be my fate.

Despite the recent weeklong hospitalization, I once again have the additional sensation of leaning against an electrified farmer's fence. Both my bladder and bowel movement are more difficult again, despite using a very low dose of opioids. I've even had to ration my very low, daily opioid dose because I do not have a new prescription yet, and the hospital has not gotten back to me. The weeklong ketamine infusion worked almost too well; having a nearly pain-free body is now a bittersweet memory instead of a daily experience.

* * *

It's October 14, 2017, and it's always a weird time because it's yet another anniversary of the skydiving accident. Sadly, I haven't seen my Navajo beau in weeks, and don't know if I still have a boyfriend, despite our daily texts, "nite nite" and "sweet dreams," replete with kissy face emoticons. We had a falling out after we spent a night at a hotel to celebrate my birthday. It was the first time we'd spent the night together, and I feared it might have been the last.

Lately I'm thinking about who I would have become without the accident. I never was an *I'm with the band* kind of girl: when my body was whole, I once refused an offer by my friend Prince to join him on a trip to Frankfurt, in his private plane. It was just a kind, platonic invitation. When I was modeling and in showbiz, there were others who were less friendly, those who wanted to trade sex with me for a proverbial backstage pass. *Yeah, I don't think so!*

I never slept or flirted with guys to get ahead in my career; I considered myself strictly a recreational, instead of a strategic fucker. By the way, doesn't the word *strategic fucker* sound a lot nicer than the derogative *gold digger*? Anyways, as a young girl, I never fantasized or longed to get married or start a family, another one of my quirks. While I unexpectedly found true love and got married, sadly, it seemed as if I never quite could open my heart and soul to my now ex-husband.

Looking back, it feels as if I have let life lead me by the nose, rather than taking charge and leading my life. Instead of solidifying a career or vocation, I had neither the confidence nor the conviction to make something wonderful out of the incredible chances that were given to me. I am not particularly proud of my life, or of myself. On the Costa Rican set of *1492: Conquest of Paradise*, Nick Gillard, the British stuntman and stunt coordinator, had told me: "You're real ugly on the inside, you know."

I was such a naïve, insecure 23 year-old fool—in love—that I just sulked instead of telling him, "Dude, haven't seen Star Wars, but had you handled your bedroom sword with as much enthusiasm as that lightsaber scene everyone raves about, we could have been dating. Schmuck!" (Honesty dictates me to admit the previous sentence is on-stage joke since it wasn't till 2017, 2018 that I found out that Nick was behind the choreography.) Sadly, then 35-year-old Nick had pointed out a sore spot: I have *always* felt ugly, on the inside and the outside. My kindness, go-getter nature, and interest in humanity never seemed to matter much either, though I tried.

Nick had been too moody to be around, so one morning I packed my dad's 1950's backpack with my belongings and a page ripped from the airline magazine, with a cartoon like depiction of Costa Rica and stuck out my thumb, hitchhiked far away from the movie set. I went mountaineering and rafting, and one evening during their strongest earthquake ever recorded, calmed down Costa Ricans who ran around hysterically instead of standing in a doorway like Angelenos had taught me. Before I left, I'd also helped the special F/X team set fire to one of the structures on the square, that was my happiest memory.

But I couldn't yet listen to my feelings, otherwise I would have known that special F/X were my forte. I still remember a warm, firm handshake at the beach with a British guy Nick introduced me to. I had to ask Nick his name, as I didn't recognize Ridley Scott and up till then, had been clueless who directed 1492. Small planet, in the early 2000's, I glanced in a mirror and saw Sigourney Weaver at a small NYC hairdresser, we were the only clients. I kept a respectful distance, but am an admirer, whether in "Alien",

"Working Girl" or "Paul" with Simon Pegg, she's a beautiful legend, equally talented as smart.

* * *

My whole life, it seems I have treated my friends, and even strangers, better than I've treated myself; I have given everyone something of me, even when my own sense of self has remained so unclear. When my family and I were lost in the mountains, when we had to hike four more hours in perilous terrain with night quickly approaching, I was the one cheering them up, so acting dapper became a second nature. My father's stress level exploded so much at times that despite the fresh mountain air, a cloud of tension could only be pierced by my laughter and antics. And I was the one targeted by that old shepherd in the mountain cabin.

I try to be a good person, but somehow, that seemed never rewarded. Perhaps, that is exactly the point: it's about finally growing up and taking charge of my life, my actions, and my future. But sadly, as always, the future remains uncertain. Perhaps one of the saddest memories I have from before my accident concerns my old buddy Prince. I was in Hamburg for a modeling job and loved dancing, so I walked over from the Pension, a cheap hotel where I was staying. Fate had placed us in the same nightclub, in the late '80s. Was I overjoyed to see an old friend? No.

Naturally, Prince, was surrounded by bodyguards and supermodels, cordoned off by a velvet rope. I didn't see his dad anywhere, and I was petrified of saying hello because I felt acutely inferior to all the beauties he was surrounded by; everyone oozed sexy confidence. Thanks to internet, I now realize he may have suffered social anxiety, like me perhaps. I should have said hello, despite feeling timid, and it makes me feel like I hadn't been a good friend. And since all we have in this life is kindness towards one another, that made me feel like a failure. But I can do better in the future, right, and become a better friend, to myself and others?

AFTERWORD

Happiness depends on ourselves. - Aristotle, Greek philosopher and scientist

Hopefully 2017 will be the last time I titled a doc, "My Suicidal Year." Then again, perhaps not. The future, as always, is uncertain. For everyone. How did I cope with this year, and the preceding year's events and battles? Sometimes, for weeks and months, I had no caregiver, they'd just disappear or moved to another agency, after a few times. And yet, some surprised me by braiding my hair, working hard, and hanging an aerial yoga hammock.

The longer I am incapacitated and bedridden, the fewer friends visit, and it seems hard to make new ones without a job or a social network. It's understandable that some friends have disappeared into the shadows, as our circumstances have changed. It can't be easy to see someone suffer, and despite my easy smile, I'm obdurate and can be a tad difficult. But my existence is akin to living in purgatory.

I feel overwhelmed on a daily basis, yet something has shifted. Since the weeklong hospitalization for ketamine, I am *finally* prioritizing my body as never before, even if I've had some huge setbacks recently. That's bound to happen, but overall, I no longer throw my energy away at frivolous stuff. I try to treat my body and mind as if I matter, the way I'd take care of a beloved friend. I have changed, and the priorities sort themselves out.

Paradoxically, despite feelings of intense loneliness, there has been an upside to fewer people visiting. Having no caregivers has turned out to be a blessing. Yes, my body has suffered for it; I have more back spasms since sitting on my upholstered bar stool, slowly unloading and loading the dishwasher. I'm learning to rest between and even during tasks, pacing, so the dishwasher takes me two days. I can't vacuum, and doing laundry takes me weeks. Walking, standing and especially sitting hurt, yet not having to deal with another human in my space, is unexpectedly wonderful.

* * *

Oh, how I wished for this book to have a more auspicious ending, but this

is life. I am content. I carry this lightness about me, and yet, I finally feel
grounded, at home with myself, so that everything around me does not matter
as much. How can someone like me, an adventurer and world traveler, live in
this limited life and body? Perhaps because I have tapped into what makes
me intrinsically happy: the courage to keep writing and performing comedy. I
wrote and published on *Medium*, and they've been well-received.

And maybe one day, I will have the confidence to record some funny
monologues from my hospital bed and post them on YouTube. I'm scared to
put myself online and for others to see me, seemingly doing nothing. But I
oughtn't feel as if I have anything to hide. I just never want anyone to think I
am lazy, lying in bed all day as a grown-ass woman. It's a bit embarrassing.
But, so what? What do I care what other people think? They don't have
adhesive arachnoiditis, intractable or chronic pain.

Slowly but surely, even memories from childhood are becoming more
vivid and outrageous under my comedic eye. It is as if everything I needed
for happiness and comedy was right here all along. Fifteen years ago, my
sister encouraged me to write a book about my adventures, culminating in my
marriage and Physician Assistant degree. Nicolien thought that was an
incredibly happy ending to a peculiar life. How wrong we were because it is
today, this moment, writing in my hospital bed in a small downtown studio,
listening to my beloved Miriam Makeba, that I am most me.

So, this is my strange and happy-ish ending; thanks to the ketamine
infusions, I exercise three times a week, write, perform comedy, and most
importantly, live alone with occasional help from friends. Weirdly, I am
gutsier than ever and certainly have more mental strength than when I was
younger. What I do, taking my power wheelchair and maimed body to the
gym, performing a show or an open mic, is way harder, and surely much
more courageous than skydiving or ice climbing.

I've also found my voice, although I'm working on not to getting mad at
fucktwats. It is not easy. I spend between 15 and 20 hours a week on phone
calls pertaining to medical administration, investigating my options, dealing
with insurers, city administrators, and my fight for a better quality of life. It
took me years, but I slowly downscaled my home, simplified my life and of
course, sold my minivan, which helped pay for my outpatient ketamine
infusions.

* * *

Strangely, I didn't shed a tear when Prince died, or Bowie, no matter how brilliant they were. But I cried for hours after Tony Scott, Ridley Scott's talented brother, leapt to his death at night, from a bridge in 2012. I knew what it was like to fall to your death, and had Tony been offered ketamine that could have made a difference—or not, he may have suffered a terminal disease. Be that as it may, then why not die surrounded by your loved ones, like in the 2003 must-see movie *The Barbarian Invasion*, via physician assisted death? Their production company, Scott Free, alludes to 'without suffering injury or punishment.'

As humans we are programmed, through evolution, to see patterns, and so the Scott brothers occupy a little more than the normal space of neurons in my brain. Not only because of Tony Scott's death, but my friend Charlie and I had seen *Blade Runner, The Director's Cut*, the evening before my skydiving accident, on October 9, 1992. There will always be a before and after accident, until I die. The morning after the accident in the ICU, I already knew that one day in the future, I would be twice the age I was when my parachute malfunctioned. I could see my fate all the way up to the moment where I'm writing in my hospital bed.

All in all, since I started ketamine therapy, my neuropathic pain has decreased, which means I'm a success story, but not fully. My severe left leg, sacral and trunk torment, and that annoying buzzing sensation are back the second I overdo things, or I am upright too long. The ketamine is not a cure as I need maintenance treatments, and ideally, I ought to have a monthly infusion (an insurmountable challenge at $950 each).

I started this book by saying, I'll give myself one more year, and now, I am too mad at Medicare to die. Also, there are too many, monumentally unanswered questions. Will I make more new friends like the fabulous Laura Johnson? Will I have fun in Arizona next February, being a special guest at my lovely gay friends' house? Will I do stand-up comedy there? Will my boyfriend and I still date? Most importantly, will my comedy improve?

* * *

my home and ears, a cacophony of sounds, of pathos, of moans, of my friends' complaining about their husbands or boyfriends, while I'm sick and done and tired one time I was afraid that if I died, there was no one to find me, now I'm just afraid death won't come quick enough to spare me the suffering

I'm always on tour. The Crippled Comedy Tour...cuz that's how I roll! One friend was like; that's so negative. Well, duh. This isn't the accessible comedy tour, or the handicapable comedy tour. Look, just accept I'm a crip, mate. Of course I'm a crip, see my dark blue sequin gown...I'm no blood, darn it!

if you have a buddy who 'broke all their bones when his parachute didn't open but he healed and traveled to Tibet and now he's fine' well, FUCK YOU do not tell me these stories, okay? And when I see you in the dressing room at the gym and you complain to me about your wrist, or knee, or ankle all the while discussing your upcoming desert hike, FUCK YOU TOO and please, quit telling me I'm such an inspiration

ladies, if he detours to buy or sell an ounce of weed and picks up a high school buddy, it's not a date

there may be no country for grumpy old men, but all sprouts locations will hire them, and they get super miffed when you loudly ask for the non-organic, normal apples

you know you've lost your caregiver's respect when she says: wished I could snuggle up under a blanket, too...my fibromyalgia is acting up

you're definitely a Dutch redneck when you're heading to a festival and realize all your gear is Coleman instead of REI, until you discover the cool hippies won't notice anyway, although problematically, they're also too stoned to build latrines

I wear yoga pants daily...they make me look way less crippled, right?

don't feel sorry for me....just because I'm an Albuquerque comic

turns out, you do need a working parachute

* * *

Never mind melancholic entries and droll observations in my comedy notebook; the hardest—and most lonesome—truth is that my skydiving accident did not teach me to value the finite length of life. Instead of pursuing academic dead ends, I really should have received a Ph.D. in Failing. Who knew it was possible to make so many mistakes, in the course of a couple of decades of living? I used to be so cocky, I marveled at all the things I had survived. Falling from a three-story building in Tokyo, crashing through a corrugated plastic garage. A huge rock hurling towards me, splitting my helmet in two, when I was conquering a frozen waterfall. Jumping from a four-story structure onto a giant air mattress. Running from a huge snow avalanche as a nine-year old.

Racing through the Dutch woods as a stunt driver for a TV show. Fracturing my left ankle in 1991 when another car stunt went awry. A week before my parachute failed, while riding on my 250cc Honda Rebel on Pico Boulevard after dark, a driver rolled down his window and yelled, "You're gonna get into an accident, you gotta be careful!" I didn't take advice from Los Angeles drivers serious: a few days before buying the Honda Rebel I relied on public transportation and someone, a friendly stranger, gave me a ride. *Wow*, I thought, *Angelenos are friendly*, but then he offered me $25 for a blowjob. I escaped at a traffic light, laughing at my near brushes with death, and fate.

For decades, I've avoided asking myself the hardest question of all: why *did* my accident happen? Mistakes were made, by me, but definitely by Skydive Perris. My altimeter was taped off at the 1000 feet mark; conceivably, first-time night skydivers oughtn't be instructed to open at 2500 if they usually open at 3500 feet. The day after I came to at Riverside General, my altimeter's glowstick disappeared which annihilated any evidence. Jumpmaster Dave had taken the device up for a skydive, to 'evaluate for malfunction.' The Dutch don't sue, and my parents discouraged me. I believed it had been my fault anyways and didn't listen to anyone who argued: "Are you sure about not filling a lawsuit, what if you worsen in 20 years?"

For years tortured myself, wishing my face had been taken, instead of my legs. I've never had much use for my face. Sigh. For now, the pounding muscle in my rib cage keeps my body going. And that injured chest, filled with grief, seems to be healing, decades after the rib fractures and that horrifying night in the desert. This is the hand I was dealt. This is my reality. And I have a lot to be thankful for, even if my life, itself, will never again be *free* by what I used to consider *normal* standards.

There isn't a day when I am not confronted with my body's limitations. Yet, I live on my own, and through comedy, finally found my voice. And that is no small feat. Throughout my life, I have been obdurate, gregarious, and wrong as many times as I've been right. Although, if I'm honest, I've probably been more wrong than right. In the end, it comes down to this: I have lived, and I have apologized. I was loved, and I have loved. I was, and am, still here.

PART FOUR

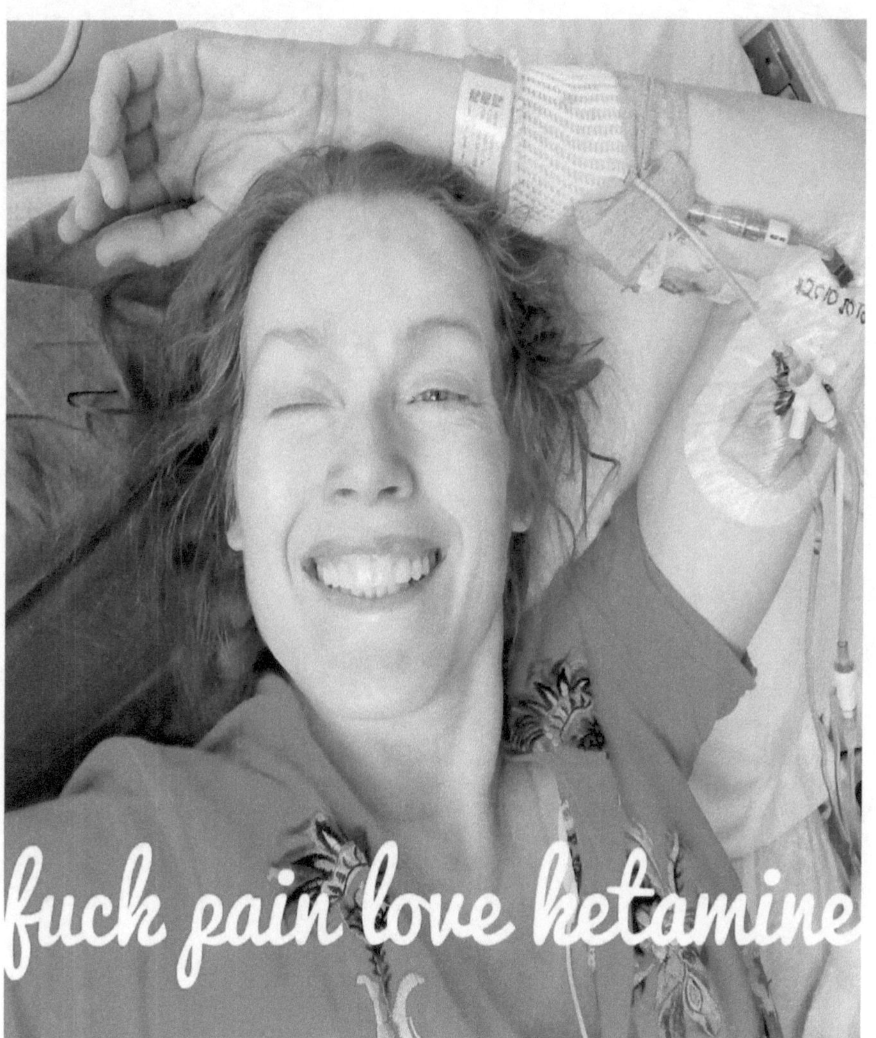

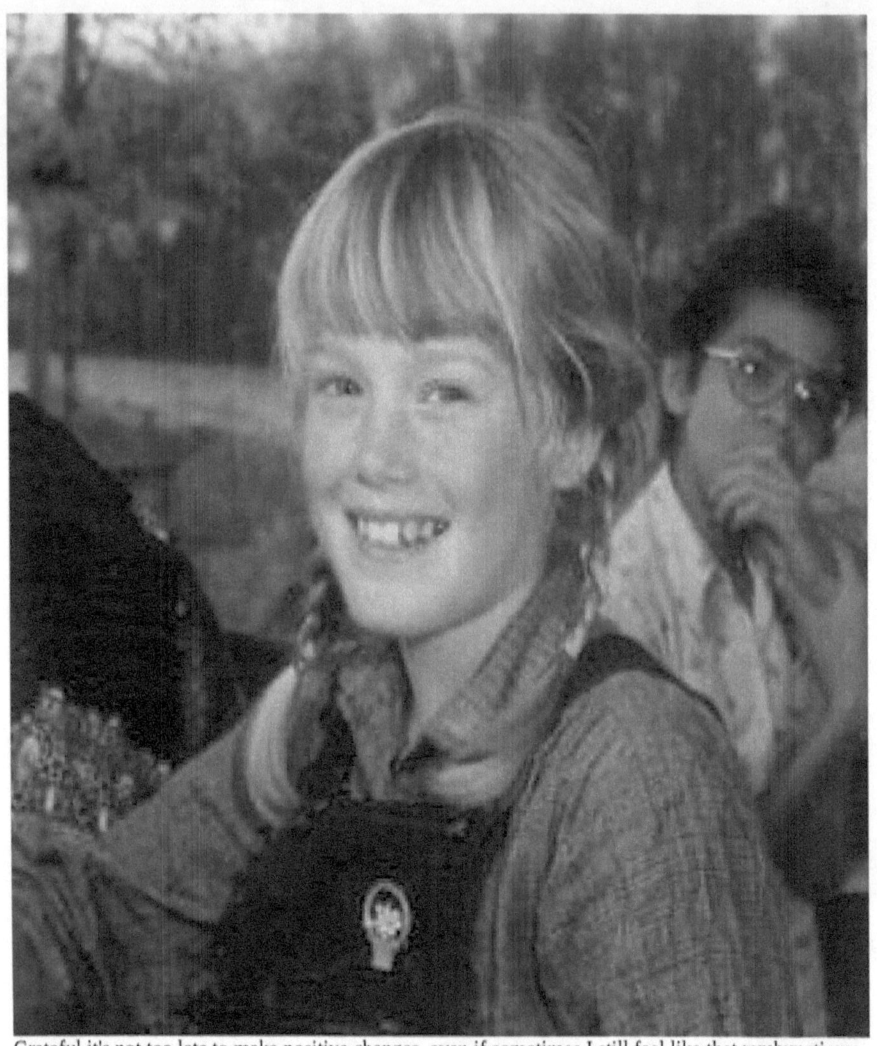

Grateful it's not too late to make positive changes, even if sometimes I still feel like that rambunctious, yet gregarious 10 year-old at Rainbow Elementary. Note the wolf teeth, and Marco behind me.

PRACTICAL ADVICE

Living with Chronic Pain, CRPS, Spinal Cord Injuries, Adhesive Arachnoiditis and/or Other Chronic Physical or Psychiatric Illness

Be Gentle

The most important thing: don't overdo it yet stay physically as active as possible. Facebook and Instagram pictures of home improvement, wheelchair basketball, and other adaptive sports get a lot of likes. The downside is osteoarthritis. For example, our shoulder joints are not a replacement for hip joints. Patients who use a wheelchair daily for decades may end up with severe bilateral shoulder osteoarthritis in their fifties and sixties, some even requiring a shoulder joint replacement.

Years of walking with a cane in my right hand, an uneven gait, and carrying a heavy bag with groceries in my left hand means the left shoulder joint has chronic bursitis. These issues did not improve with manual wheelchair use, although swimming and OT/PT stretches have helped immensely. One of the biggest blind spots in the medical/therapeutic field is that when we are young and newly injured, aging is never discussed, nor are we recommended *gentle* exercise, especially with an incomplete spinal cord injury or adhesive arachnoiditis. Our bodies may appear outwardly normal yet pose significant challenges.

Try and rest at least an hour a day, without distractions from your smartphone. Recharge your batteries in the middle of the day, listen to a mind-body recording such as Jon Kabat-Zinn's guided meditation, nap, take a bath, anything that will help you relax. Some Physical/Occupational Therapists have a hard time with neuropathic pain and adhesive arachnoiditis. You can't blame them, they've never heard of it. If you are referred for PT or OT, show Dr. Tennant's recommendations, and focus on *gently* stretching the spine and spinal roots, to avoid further injuries. Bring up nerve gliding technique, this may be instrumental in helping neck, shoulder and leg pain.

Medical Records

Keep all records in a binder with tabs, include discs with MRIs/CT scans. This is a separate binder from medical bills and insurance. It ought to contain all your lab work, follow-ups, letters from medical providers, radiology, and other reports. Use tabs for specialists, and keep a few blank sheets to jot down questions, notes, and dates for phone calls. Have one sheet with all your primary care and specialists' phone numbers.

Be careful who you loan out your MRI discs to; years ago, a Lovelace physician borrowed my discs to present my "interesting" case, and despite multiple attempts to get them back, I didn't. A lot of hospitals and clinics provide patient portals. These are terrific for making appointments or asking your medical team a question. Make sure you have Power of Attorney and Health Directives ready as needed.

Exercise

Do the workout that works for you. You're the expert on your body, through trial and error you will find what that workout is. If possible, elevate your heart rate, a few times a week. Hydrotherapy has been wonderful, I do use water shoes to alleviate the allodynia from touching the pool floor with bare feet. The shoes are lightweight yet sturdy, as I cannot walk or even stand bare foot, with atrophied, painful feet. The shoes I like are on Amazon, they will last you at least a year. I use silicone earplugs to make my swim even more quiet, especially when people chat loudly, or the hot tub is on. Water shoes and silicone earplugs are listed under Kaatje's Favorite Things in Resources.

Find a simple, effective workout you can do from home, or at a gym at least three times a week. The key is moderation—and a convenient location. If your yoga class is too far away, or the exercises are too strenuous, your body will suffer. It may not be a possible solution for everyone, but I moved to a downtown studio apartment, and use my power wheelchair to independently reach a heated, small and quiet pool, five minutes away. Because my body's thermostat was completely disintegrated by 2014/2015, I could no longer swim in a public pool; the water is too cold. Although I will swim despite a 9-level agony: it may as if my sacrum and left leg are on fire, but swimming and gentle movement decreases the suffering to a 7 or 8, sometimes a 6.

Adapt, if possible. I do a *sitting warrior* pose from my wheelchair pillow, and mimic *standing tree* while lying down. Again, don't overdo it, since that may lead to post-polio syndrome—muscle atrophy from working atrophied muscles too hard. I'm always at risk of over-exercising, however, being active three times a week has preserved my muscles, flexibility, and sanity. With adhesive arachnoiditis, there is so much bizarre, electrical pain; swimming and movement seems to help specifically with the weird, buzzing sensation—which Dr. Tennant explains as *trapped electricity*, from hampered cerebrospinal fluid circulation.

Even if it isn't the same as solo hiking, swimming provides happiness and sense of wellbeing. I finally know that I deserve peaceful *me* time. What's been a life saver too is always having my silicone support pillow on me, whether in the manual or power wheelchair. I place it underneath me in the hot tub during my OT and PT exercises and stretches, and it works equally well in the dry and wet sauna. The BackJoy SitzRight Wedge Seat Cushion is waterproof, and Amazon's description states it may be "helpful for sciatica and coccygeal pain."[96] I even use it on top of a shower seat; my gym has an accessible shower with Rubbermaid shower seat for me, but it's more comfortable to sit on the BackJoy.

One caveat, no matter what cause, but if you are bedridden 100% of the time instead of 90% or 50%, your caregivers need to use a little bit of (warming) body oil or lotion and stretch your body passively. All of your joints need movement, daily, whether passively or actively. Find out if you qualify for dual waiver—both Medicaid and Medicare—or through your health insurance, try and obtain daily or alternating Occupational and Physical Therapy visits.

Medication Organization

Stay organized with the help of weeklong medication boxes, with three to four slots per day as needed. I have seven prescriptions, and take meds at 7 a.m., 12 noon, 4 p.m., and at bedtime. Occasionally, I forget to take my medications on time, but having three weeks' worth of prepared boxes helps me stay on track. My primary care provider and pain team prescribe baclofen, gabapentin, and lisinopril as 90-day scripts.

If your medical provider writes your regular, maintenance-type prescriptions for a three-month period, that saves you a lot of time and effort avoiding unnecessary pharmacy errands. Mail order is another good option if your mailbox is secure. Consider talking with your mail carrier or local post office to make alternative arrangements if you have concerns about your mail order medications delivery. Check if your pharmacy has an app for easy refills; evaluate for refills when you take care of your weekly medication box.

Opioids

Ask your provider for the Millennium Pharmacogenetic test.[97] Even without FDA approval, it may reveal how well you metabolize various drugs as it tests for 40 different medications, including opioids and muscle relaxants. Having this information may be highly advantageous to both you and your pain management provider. Millennium DNA testing will identify whether you are a *fast* or *poor* metabolizer for opioids, and in the current climate, it may come in handy to have this documented.

Millennium Pharmacogenetic testing is typically *not* reimbursed for physical ailments, but may be reimbursed for depression, a common side effect of chronic pain. Before you have the test done, confirm that your insurance carrier will pay for the test if it's ordered in conjunction with a—situational—depression diagnosis. Incidentally, knowing which anti-depressants work best for you may be helpful too.

My very personal recommendation is to use opioids for your worst pain, and you are the best, and *only* judge of what that feels like. I recommend this because, if your pain is intractable, you may have more benefit if you use opioids as judiciously as possible. In a future book, I may revise that opinion, but for now, using opioids sparingly has been beneficial to me.

The opioids I do take work, without having to increase my dosage, as a 'normal metabolizer.' However, my well-being would improve with Oxycontin 5 mg ER twice a day again, rather than using 2.5 mg of oxycodone IR four to six times a day. It would be so nice to sleep through the night, instead of pain waking me up at 2, 3 AM since oxycodone immediate-release only works for 3-4 hours.

Intravenous Ketamine

As mentioned previously, ketamine has a high safety profile, and the World Health Organization states ketamine is an 'essential' medication. But it has side-effects, as previously discussed. Consult with your pain management team if hospital-based infusions are right for you. If it fits within your budget, try outpatient treatments—around $750-$2200 per infusion.

Contact your insurance carrier to find out if they reimburse. The Ketamine Advocacy Network, and my Resources, are a good place to start.[98] That said, it may take quite a few phone calls to find a reasonably priced and convenient location. Most websites do not give prices outright.

In an outpatient setting, I usually receive around a total of 240 mg of ketamine over three and a half hours. As an inpatient, the dose is 65 mg per hour, around the clock and I am lying horizontal which is better in my situation. I enjoy the added magnesium to the ketamine drip as it seems to have a synergistic effect and provides longer-lasting, pain relief.[99] Temporary side effects include diplopia (double vision), visions, vivid dreams and sensations. I now call them visions, instead of hallucinations, which for me, takes the edge off the psychological side effects.

Your mind may convince you those vivid dreams or visions are real. Before the infusion starts, remind yourself these side effects are all transient. Those sensations generally cease within 15 minutes of the infusions being complete. Hold a token in your hand, like in that movie *Inception*. You can open your eyes, look at it, feel it and you'll realize you're okay, it's just a ketamine infusion in a room. That said, I saw *Inception* twice and still don't know which one was his reality!

The more ketamine infusions I had, the easier it became on my mind. After repeated treatments, I experienced much greater lucidity and even more of a reduction in terms of physical suffering. As I mentioned earlier, medications may help alleviate the side effects, and you should feel free to communicate your needs to the providers during the treatment. Although I experienced panic attacks and even a 'k-hole' on ketamine, the analgesic effect was so great, I had to keep going.

Prepare a bag that has everything you need to be comfortable. You may want to bring earplugs, one of the best brands is Moldex Pura-Fit Tapered Foam. These, and a fabulous eye mask are listed on Kaatje's Favorite Things, google Amazon or check the Resources. Definitely bring an eye mask for sleep, an eye patch for double vision, a case for your glasses, and a scarf. If it's a hospital ketamine infusion, I bring blue painter's tape for my Chromebook cords, phone charger, and other electronic devices. I pack a case for my nightguards and an electric toothbrush.

Communicate with your care team; e.g. a quiet room, a chair with a pillow next to the sink, a warm/hot/cool room temperature, door signs asking to for tempered voices and to keep the door closed. If there are a lot of windows that let in too much light, tape will hold square diaper pads to cover the windows, with the added benefit of muting noise.

By far the most important in-hospital advice is to request a *midline* IV—which has a longer catheter. Dr Rogelj strongly recommended it, and I refused. But magnesium is hard on your veins, and without a midline I ended up with three blown IVs. The moral of this story, and book? Don't be stubborn like me.

Miscellaneous, Supportive Meds for Ketamine Infusions

Whether inpatient or outpatient, before the ketamine is started, ask for Toradol (ketorolac) 30 mg IV. It's a fast-working, strong anti-inflammatory and a non-opioid pain killer. I've had some nausea and even vomiting, so now I ask for at least 6.25 or 12.5 mg of Phenergan (promethazine) before the ketamine infusion starts, or before a dose increase. It has the additional benefit of being an anti-histamine and sedative. Especially if you're doing a ketamine infusion for the first time it's nice to feel a little sleepy. Although true allergies to ketamine are rare—four case reports in 50+ years—it's a nice thing to have on-board.

Definitely discuss magnesium with your inpatient or outpatient team and bring a list of these miscellaneous meds. A lot is trial and error; during my first hospitalization I kept throwing up the day after the infusion was started. The staff administered Zofran (ondansetron) a few times, which made me feel more nauseated, given the strong chemical smell after pushing the medication through an IV line. Zofran also doesn't have Phenergan's anti-histamine and sedative properties. I urge providers and patients to consider using Phenergan as a first line medication. It's a personal preference perhaps, but Phenergan feels like a nice, safe, warm blanket.

Ketamine at Home

If you have access to a compounding pharmacy, your pain management physician or primary care provider can prescribe ketamine either as a nasal spray or 'troches.' (Troches dissolve between your gums and cheeks.) Ketamine prescriptions can be given over the phone and allow for refills. Some pharmacies can even mail you the medication in a padded envelop. As a compounded medication, with the racemic mixture, the prescriptions are as follows—note, I stopped using the intranasal spray and switched to troches:

- For the nasal spray: "Instill 1 or 2 sprays in each nostril 1 to 3

times daily as needed for pain, 50 mg/ml, 15 ml." A nearby compounding pharmacy charges $49.99—around $25 a month, with one spray in each nostril daily before bedtime.
- For the troches: "Ketamine 75 mg troches. Dissolve 1 troche in mouth between gum and cheek every 8 to 12 hours, for 30 days. Quantity 90." Cost: $90.

The compounding pharmacy that manufactures my troches is 40 minutes away yet it's facility cannot manufacture a nasal spray, whereas a nearby compounding pharmacy produces both nasal spray and troches but charges over $40 more for the troches. Research backs me up; for some people IV, intranasal or oral seems to work better, and sometimes different doses of the same route. It's trial and error.

You may find that troches work better than nasal spray, even if it usually is the other way around. Experiment with using ¼ of a troche around two to three times a day. I break the troche in half, then flatten the troche paste and gently pull it apart so I am really only taking a quarter, around 19 mg. It's still not cheap on a fixed income but spending around $20-25 a month on something that works, immediately, seems like a good deal.

If the nasal spray works, and you use one spray in each nostril daily, each bottle will last you about two months. I switched to troches as they seem more effective for my pain. By now you know I trust older, well tested medications that are usually more affordable. Since finishing this manuscript, an *esketamine* nasal spray was developed by Johnson and Johnson.

The Spravato nasal spray for depression, at 28 mg/ml for 2 ml, is around $624 for a supply of 2 sprays, depending on the pharmacy. Compare that with my compounded pharmacy's *racemic mixture* nasal spray, $49.99 for 50 mg/ml, with 15 ml of medication.

Vitamins

Keep it simple. Vitamin pills are large, and as a GI provider, I have seen too many patients with vitamin-induced esophagitis—inflammation of the esophageal lining—especially in aging patients. I take Vit. D because labs showed my levels were low, but I don't take a multivitamin.[100]

In my view, there isn't enough evidence to support supplemental vitamins unless you have a B12 shortage or scurvy—a Vit. C deficiency—and yes, scurvy is making a comeback in the US. I do use supplemental magnesium for the muscle spasms and bowel problems related to the spinal cord injury, and because my age justifies taking calcium citrate with the Vit D.

If I could be bothered to repeat the bone density and Vit D level tests, I'll stop the supplements if those exams are normal. You have my word. There are a lot of internet horror stories, mostly coming from the complementary and alternative medicine perspective, about so-called MTHFR deficiency—which I have too.

Pay it no mind, at least for now. As chronic patients, we have enough to worry about. One step at a time. Dr. Forest Tennant has an extensive regimen that includes a lot of supplements. I have mixed feelings about this and may explore the topic further in the next book. Last but not least: CBD. It doesn't work for me, and it's expensive.

Exhaustion

Fatigue, specifically the kind that knocks you out is a very real side effect of chronic pain. Overwhelming fatigue can happen because your body is exhausted from dealing with pain. Sometimes the fatigue is as debilitating as the illness itself. Understandably, preparing food is hard with both pain and debilitating fatigue, especially when you live alone without help or caregiving. However, my pharmacist/clinician believes some of the post-exertional fatigue may be linked to depleted glycogen, so I now eat a banana or yogurt before my swim, which helps a little.

I went from eating gummi worms or a coconut ice cream bar daily, but now, prepare a carrot/sweet potato/beans/brown rice stew, seasoned with green curry paste or laced with turmeric, cumin, coriander and ginger, which lasts me a week. I eat a mostly plant-based diet with salad, yogurt, muesli, fruits, and vegetables daily. In my opinion, the bio-industry doesn't treat animals well, so I drink almond milk. Occasionally I'll eat a pint of Häagen-Dazs or a small bag of LAY'S® Limón potato chips, but it is an exception, not the rule.

I do not believe in being paranoid about your food, yet plant-based eating, and having groceries delivered via Instacart has made a huge, positive difference. Chew your food well and eat smaller meals throughout the day to avoid esophageal and heartburn problems. Lastly, don't bother obsessing about BMI, but instead focus on nurturing a healthy body with a stable weight.

Relationships

If you have a severe illness in your forties, you either die or you recover. Staying sick means living in purgatory. I found out quickly that more than half of people I knew stopped visiting and no longer help with errands and groceries. It is normal, our lives diverged, and it can be hard to see a friend suffer.

Maybe we just didn't have enough in common anymore, and of course, friends in their forties may have young kids, or aging parents already requiring—medical—attention. That said, your heart may break from despair, loneliness, and having lost your sense of purpose in life. Still, don't be afraid to break off a friendship that no longer works.

Being chronically ill, whether physically or mentally, seems a lonely and lonesome endeavor. And yet, although I frequently feel lonely, having fewer friends means more time and energy for writing and stand-up comedy. Unfortunately, couples with a disabled partner have a higher divorce rate. My own marriage did not survive, a mixed blessing, as I never would have become a comedian or author. However, if you enjoy being married, take proactive steps! I will certainly explore this topic in another memoir.

Ultimately, as patients we must try to be self-reliant but don't forget, it is okay to seek help. Cognitive behavioral therapy, and a passion for comedy, have been the most useful support systems—although not without some abject failures on my part. Find out what provides you contentment; volunteer, interact with Facebook groups, become advocates, adopt a pet or therapy dog, all of which can provide comfort and companionship. It is of the utmost importance to find meaning, and connection, in your life. Your survival depends on it.

Home Modification

Ideally, your home should work for you, instead of the other way around. Create a simple, practical layout so cleaning up is easier, especially if a home health caregiver, a friend, or family members help you. Clutter creates more opportunity to stumble and fall, especially if you have heaps of equipment like wheelchairs, walkers, leg braces, and more. For better sleep, an electrical hospital bed seems best, or any electrical bed that can elevate the head and feet separately at the touch of a button.

I installed a Moen grab bar—a combined toilet roll holder and grab bar— and kitchen cabinets with drawers that help with my particular needs. I live in a small, accessible studio with ample space for a power wheelchair, a manual wheelchair, and a walker. Other patients have mentioned "smart" light bulbs and switches that can be turned on and off via Alexa, Google Assistant, or a Wi-Fi app. Roomba vacuums seem helpful for some people. Before I was prescribed a hospital bed, I used a Jobri Spine Reliever Bed Wedge (Google Pay) and Restorology Elevating Foam Leg Rest Pillow (Amazon). This seemed to alleviate the sacral and low back pain.

Energy

My time limit for writing is around an hour, in my hospital bed, with positional changes. After that, my tailbone hurts too much, and my brain shuts down. My limit for sitting upright is 20 minutes, yet I'll chat too much and forget to check in with my body. I'm experimenting with a timer because I need to avoid flare-ups. It's the same for too much texting and writing of emails. Find out what your own limit is, whether it is 30 or 300 steps, one or two phone calls, or 20 texts daily. Stick to your own boundaries for a few weeks to see if that helps.

Take frequent breaks in positioning, I use a 30-minute timer for writing, then I force myself to stretch or make a cup of tea. However, some aggravating factors cannot be avoided at times; like writing this book required way more energy than I have, and when stuff goes awry, the amount of phone calls and emailing has taken a real physical toll. I'm learning to accept that I cannot always keep my pain to a minimum or exist within my boundaries, but I am slowly improving in that regard.

Simplify Your Life

It took me over two decades to get my life decluttered, and I'm still not there. I started out great, by donating my old ice climbing pickaxes and boots to the local climbing group. That was a great start. But various major events led me to clear out too hastily and too quickly, which left me filled with regret and grief, years later. I often have let go of stuff out of anger. Trust me, that's not the way to do it.

Letting go of stuff is great, but if you don't have something to replace it with, like a new hobby, you may end up feeling emptier, and sadder.

Marie Kendo has great decluttering and organizational tips, check out her own website, or this easy guide to get started.[101] Although it is true that we all probably own too much, it is preferable to say goodbye to material things in a better mood. The best thing about donation, recycling, or selling stuff is that you'll have more energy because you won't ever again need to search for items you no longer possess.

Downsize your home and live in a one-story or a one-floor apartment if that is feasible. Slowly grow towards a pragmatic state of mind. My downfall will always be too many DIY projects, but I've made some progress on that front.

Speaking of simplifying: a Mirena IUD has been a life saver since 2008. There is enough bowel and bladder care to deal with, I love not having to bother with tampons or pads. IUDs are mainly used for contraception but they're very useful for people with health issues. I had an IUD even when I didn't have sex. A few years ago, I was in between IUDs, and had my periods once or twice: the additional back pain and cramps threw me over the edge. If you suffer from longstanding health issues, consider taking menstruation out of the equation completely.

Neuropathic Pain & Neurogenic Bladder/Bowel

A simple, yet profound and effective remedy: ice packs. Target sells the best; *look for reusable cold + hot gel pack.* The ingredients of cold packs have changed, and they don't seem as good as a few years ago. Still, those Target gel ice packs are highly effective to trick your mind into thinking the lower half of your body is not on fire, by placing them on your sacrum or low back. I use two in a large freezer bag. I've used a large block of ice as well, but that caused freezer burns.

Anti-seizure medications like gabapentin (Neurontin) or pregabalin (Lyrica) may alleviate pain. Trial and error will tell if they work for you. I'm a big fan of acetazolamide (Diamox) for neuroinflammation, at 375 mg (250 mg tablets, I take 1.5 daily). Unfortunately, as you now know, neuropathic pain is hard to treat, and yet it's a huge problem in the US: there are 14 million individuals with diabetes, and a quarter of them have painful diabetic neuropathy. Research indicates pregabalin works quicker than gabapentin and is a more potent analgesic as well. I was on gabapentin, then switched to pregabalin for a few years.[102] In the end, gabapentin suited me better.

I tend to trust medications that have been around for much longer; gabapentin has been on the market for 25-30 years. Side effects of sleepiness went away with prolonged use and by slowly increasing the dose. Start low, go slow. I added amitriptyline at night, a tricyclic anti-depressant invented during the 1950s. For me, amitriptyline's side effects of dry mouth worsened significantly at 75 mg BID, and I cut back down to one 75 mg tablet, at night.

We've gone over this earlier; hyperalgia, allodynia, and burning, electrical pain sensations relate to neuropathic pain. The excellent, concise book *Neuropathic Pain* by Oxford Pain Management Library is probably the best book on neuropathy.[103] Even if it does not mention adhesive arachnoiditis— very few books do—it explains neuropathic pain, its' multiple causes and medications to try. *Neuropathic Pain* mentions that 20-35% of patients with back pain have associated neuropathic pain, a number so astonishingly high you'd think it would have made its way to mainstream media.

Because it's a resource for medical providers, it is a bit harder to read, but so worth it. Any patient with neuropathic pain ought to skim a copy, if anything to discuss further options for treatment with your primary care provider. My copy was on Amazon for $3.74 (like new), depending on inventory.[104] You can also find it at Barnes and Nobles and other outlets, and it's listed in Kaatje's Favorite Things on Amazon. Quick reminder that if you suspect your neuropathic pain is related to adhesive arachnoiditis, read Dr. Aldrete's "Suspecting and Diagnosing Adhesive Arachnoiditis."[105]

If you can, consult with a neurologist or a rehabilitation specialist if you have mobility challenges, and ask for an ASIA (American Spinal Injury Association) neurologic exam, which tests deficits for motor, sensory nerves, and reflexes. Based on that exam, you may receive support, in the form of a referral for rehabilitation or for bladder and bowel care needs. Some patients may need a bowel and/or bladder regimen like that of SCI patients.

One of the best books is Gut: The Inside Story of Our Body's Most Underrated Organ, written by German internist Giulia Enders, her sister Jill illustrated this phenomenal book (see Kaatje's Favorite Things in Resources and/or this footnote).[106] *Gut* imbues the reader with the kind of advice I used to give my Gastroenterology patients, and yet this book that taught *me* how to improve my bowel and bladder care. This book is really helpful for most patients with neurogenic bowel and bladder, from complete and incomplete spinal cord injuries, adhesive arachnoiditis or cauda equina syndrome. And if you're on opioid pain medications, your bowels will also thank you for reading this book, as you may require extra fiber, and daily polyethylene glycol (generic Miralax) to combat constipation.

Don't waste your money on a *Potty* by the way; a Sterilite box that's 11.5 (l) x 7.5 (w) x 4.5 (h) does the trick and you can store gloves, moist wipes and other supplies. The very best advice I can give you: lean forward to mimic squatting for easier defecation, feet on the box. Add fiber, and if needed, daily, generic Mira-Lax. For neurogenic (or 'floppy') bladder: catherization or pushing down on your abdomen near your bladder with your hand may facilitate urination. Sitting in a squatting position with the box will also help with urination.

Sexuality

Well, by now you know more than my therapist about my sex-life. But what about yours? Seriously, I hope you will have an opportunity to enjoy yourself, and have fun, with or without sex, with or without a partner. Even if it's different than before your injuries and/or pain, the biggest sex organ is still your brain. It's not easy, but talk with your partner, spouse or lover what you need and want.

Rehabilitation physicians in the Netherlands are a hoot: I wasn't ready to date, let alone even contemplate sex for years after my divorce. Out of the blue my very handsome physician casually noted "You can always talk with a urology nurse about your sexual needs, and tools such as dildos." He said it with a straight face, with the medical assistant in a room. Haha only in Holland.

All kidding aside, I wished all medical providers would address sexuality more often, not just in the context of spinal cord injuries. After my skydiving accident, as a Dutch rehabilitation patient, I'd received proper education and lectures. Then, as a rehabilitation PA in the UK, we were expected to address sexuality with every one of our patients. As noted above; European, specialized nurses provide much needed support for urology and sexuality concerns.

Of course, serious disease and disorders will radically change your sexuality and confidence. But touch, intimacy and connection are an integral part of what it means to be human, yet is hardly addressed in the US medical system. Pain questionnaires during a clinic visit always ask: what makes the pain better? Ketamine, swimming and sex—preferably all on the same day, has been my standard answer the last few years!

You may find that different parts of your body respond to touch, so explore away. My face, neck and chest have become more sensitive, even if the genitourinary area has numbness. I hear of couples who haven't had sex or any physical intimacy for ten or twenty years because of physical illness or other reasons. Although understandable, it's also a bit sad. The good news is that lack of intimacy is not irreversible, it requires communication and patience.

Luckily there are so many ways to feel close and intimate, it doesn't have to be penetration or sex. It took me most of my life to learn that connection, and intimacy in whatever form, can be wonderful, human experiences. So, explore, if needed, read up on getting it on and most of all, have fun. If you are going to have sex though, don't forget protection, no matter what age.

Invasive Procedures

If you happen to suffer from adhesive arachnoiditis, or other neuropathies, I suggest that, if you can, avoid spinal cord stimulators, stem cell treatments, epidural steroidal injections, rhizotomy, or back surgery. You may not always have a choice, especially when it is a matter of life and death, or such a bad herniation that it could cause complete paralysis, bladder and bowel dysfunction, or cauda equina syndrome.[107] Nevertheless, if it is not emergency surgery, request a second opinion.

Many patients with Failed Back Surgical Syndrome may have, or are at risk for arachnoiditis, which is not helped by another surgery. The satisfaction rate after surgery is comparable to that of doing cognitive therapy paired with functional restorative medicine (dedicated exercise within a multimodal setting).[108] I am apprehensive about the future because we're looking at an epidemic of adhesive arachnoiditis patients in the next few decades. It's the perfect storm; invasive procedures have soared, especially since the CDC Opioid Guidelines came out, and patients who have had back surgeries in their thirties, forties, and fifties are now aging.

For anyone with back pain, whether mild, moderate or severe, I strongly recommend *Crooked: Outwitting the Back-Pain Industry and Getting on the Road to Recovery* by investigative writer (and back pain sufferer) Cathryn Jakobson Ramin.[109] It's one of the better books on backpain, and one of the few, who mentions adhesive arachnoiditis—in this case study, caused by epidural steroidal injections. Cathryn Jakobson Ramin: "One result is 'adhesive arachnoiditis,' a condition so grossly debilitating that neurologist Dewey Nelson described it as akin to 'having a blowtorch up your rectum. It binds the nerves, like gunky cooked spaghetti, and the result is unrelenting pain that may last for a lifetime.'"

Wow, *having a blowtorch up your rectum* sounds exactly like adhesive arachnoiditis! The scope of this book and memoir does not allow me to delve deeply into each invasive procedure, but please. Be cautious. Investigate the pros and cons of every invasive treatment, including stem cells. Understand that 10% of spinal surgeries for lumbar fusions were not medically indicated. This doesn't just constitute Medicare fraud, it puts patients at risk.[110]

There is no issue more divisive in on-line communities with intractable pain, or rare diseases, than that of stem cell treatment. The desperation is great; there are people with end-stage pulmonary fibrosis who are dying, right now. For every research success a University lab posts via press release, the comment sections are filled with hundreds of heartbroken, suffering lung patients wanting to enroll in a trial, that was done on *rats*.

Compare your stem cell doctor's website to that of stem cell researchers and scientists. Many stem cell clinics do not have the decades of experience that would enable them to safely provide stem cell treatment. Frequently, *autologous* stem cells are advertised for a wide variety of illnesses such as adhesive arachnoiditis, erectile dysfunction, and Parkinson's—this is a red flag, one treatment that claims to treat a variety of complex ailments. Autologous means material harvested from the patient themselves, for example adult fat cells.

Some commercial stem cell clinics provide a "Pay-to-Participate Phase 1 clinical trial" although they've never published the research. In a Pay-to-Participate trial, the patient pays for treatment, which is not considered ethical by stem cell scientists. Patients are told that stem cells may take "up to 18 months to start working," which seems questionable. Chronic diseases are cyclical; they vary from day to day, month to month, year to year; fluctuations may not correlate to stem cell treatment. Some patients complain their symptoms have aggravated, since stem cell treatment. Other patients' spinal cords became infected after treatment with umbilical stem cells.[111]

Dr. Paul Knoepfler's website and the California Institute for Regenerative Medicine (CIRM) explain stem cell treatment, trials and the science on their websites, in more detail than I can provide in this book.[112] [113] Neuropathic pain is a nightmare, so I understand the appeal of stem cell treatments. After all, I tried DMT, *The Spirit Molecule*, out of desperation, so I'm the last to judge you. As patients with severe and often intractable pain—and a blow torch up our rectum—we are facing incredible odds. How do we make the right decisions for our healthcare and pain management?

It *is* really confusing. Pay-to-participate stem cell trials appear on the clinicaltrial.gov website (via a loophole), while the FDA simultaneously warns patients to avoid unregulated and non-FDA approved stem cell treatments.[114] Inform yourself of the benefits and also the risks, of all invasive procedures. Understand that glowing reviews of stem cell treatment are testimonials, until well designed clinical trials determine proven efficacy and safety. Stem cell treatments are not reimbursed by insurers, but inpatient ketamine infusions are, at least by some Medicare/Medicaid insurers.

Consumer Reports wrote an excellent article on stem cell treatment, reiterating that scientific research is promising, but that the benefit of autologous stem cells is questionable.[115] There are other concerns: if you underwent stem cell treatment by a private clinic, that excludes you from participating in FDA sanctioned Phase 2 or 3 clinical trials.

Compare commercial websites to that of The Tisch MS Research Center of NY.[116] Reputable research centers will be *transparent*: "Our Phase I study began in 2014, 20 patients were enrolled, and all 20 patients received 3 treatments of mesenchymal stem cell neural progenitors (MSC-NPs) [...] In addition to proving MSC-NP treatment to be safe [....] the FDA gave Tisch MSRCNY the greenlight to go ahead with our plans for Phase II. Phase II will consist of 50 patients receiving stem cells in a placebo-controlled double-blind study."[117]

Although serious stem cell research is promising, this has not yet translated into medical applications performed by reputable clinics and hospitals—except for leukemia, lymphoma and certain patients with burns. [118] I believe we're about 10+ years away from clinical applications, for adhesive arachnoiditis even longer as it's an underdiagnosed disease. E.g., the National MS Society was included in a pilot project to find out how many people have MS in the United States.[119]

This turned out to be 1 million, more than twice the number expected. I am positive adhesive arachnoiditis shows similar numbers, but without a national network and funding, tough luck. Lastly, I emphasize with the desire for hope, or a cure, and if I ever change my mind, you will be the first to know. I already sold my car and then my home, to pay for outpatient ketamine infusions and medical expenses, which added up to $23,000 over the years 2016-2019—this includes the $1575 copayment for each hospitalization. Had I believed that stem cells could have alleviated the neurological pain, I would have done so.

Miscellaneous

Don't neglect dental health and vaccinations. Brush your teeth with an electric toothbrush, if possible, and floss daily. It saves on energy, too. I rinse with generic *Biotene* dry mouth rinse from Walmart, then floss at night. See your dentist at least once a year, and your dental hygienist for cleanings, especially if you use medications that may affect your gum health, such as dry mouth or gingival hyperplasia (inflamed gums from anti-seizure meds). Get a bone density test.

Treat yourself and your family to an annual flu shot, pneumonia, and other applicable vaccines, such as shingles. Have hormones tested as chronic pain may cause low blood levels. In general, try and set up a care system with friends, family, or caregivers. Make sure someone has an extra key to your home. Get your finances in order, decide on a living will, set up advanced directives, and complete other important paperwork.

Read Dr. Forrest Tenant's websites, books, protocols, and articles, as he is one of the few physicians, who specialized in both pain management and adhesive arachnoiditis. Unfortunately, his treatment of thousands of patients did not result in a consensus statement across the nation. However, Dr. Tenant has been a relentless advocate for patients with this chronic disease, and he currently serves as Editor Emeritus for *Practical Pain Management,* a great source for patients with adhesive arachnoiditis and/or other chronic pain (see Resources, to which I added his books on Amazon).

Loneliness

Living in solitary confinement is, in truth, one of the worst things that could result from your chronic pain condition.[120] I have no family in the USA, and although I do have a couple of friends, recently when the hospital phoned to say they had a bed available for another weeklong ketamine infusion, early 2018, I could not go. Why? I was in too much pain to pack a bag and take the bus to the Rio Grande Hospital by myself. The very kind nurse asked, "Is there anyone you can call to help?" "No," I replied softly.

And often I do not want help. Friends are wonderful, the few I have in my life, but they're also exhausting when I do not enforce my own boundaries. For instance, if I tell a friend I can only visit for thirty minutes, but I do not tell my visitors it's time for them to leave, I often end up dishonoring my own limits. The isolating nature of a serious chronic condition is a battle that I'm finally learning to cope with. But it will never be easy. Just know that feeling isolated can be a huge part of the disease.[121] I sometimes choke on my loneliness, and I will say yes to an "opportunity" because I yearn for human contact. However, the more I learn to live within my boundaries, the happier I became.

I recommend waiting to accept an invitation until you're sure you're up for it, rather than hastily agreeing, especially if your motives are solely to remedy your loneliness. One of my essays on *Medium* is titled, "On Being Bedbound," and another "Why I Abandoned All Hope." Ironically, writing those essays gave me hope.[122]

Online Support

Online networks can provide much-needed support through Facebook and/or patient advocacy groups. Internet delivers products such as non-perishable groceries (through Amazon or Walmart), and even amazing, comfortable clothes via Stitch Fix or ASOS.com. Ordering groceries online through Instacart, paying bills and having online banking have a profound, positive impact on my life.

In the Resources section, you'll find helpful Facebook groups and other websites that are a wealth of information, especially if you are newly diagnosed with adhesive arachnoiditis, central neuropathic pain syndrome, or neuropathy. One of the most informative and compassionate websites out there, as many neuropathies seem to overlap, is the Reflex Sympathetic Dystrophy Syndrome Association—RSDSA.

Their mission statement: *To provide support, education, and hope to all affected by the pain and disability of CRPS/RSD, while we drive research to develop better treatments and a cure.* RSDSA is an effective patient- and research driven organization, with a $2.2 million operating budget and must-read articles such as "Methods for Minimizing Pain Flares."[123]

Jim Broatch, RSDSA Executive Vice President and Director stated, via personal communication: "Since 1992 we spend $2.7 million on research, although our operating budget is divided between patients and research, they each get 50%. Our research has one criteria: what brings the most relief to patients right now. We have a 20-year longitudinal study, how CRPS affects health overall but results were clear; so, the study will be published 10 years sooner, in Oct 2019. We published Clinical Practice Guidelines, since 1/3 to 1/4 of patients who do not get treated early enough will end up with disabling CRPS."[124] Jim's remarks, and the RSDSA website advice is applicable to *all* patients with neuropathies, as they will need a multi-disciplinary approach.

Sitting Disability

Some patients with low back pain, sciatica and those with sacral pain or adhesive arachnoiditis complain of an abject inability to sit. A sitting disability is terrifying; I dragged pillows everywhere, but I also couldn't stand for more than a few minutes. It's hard to fathom how complicated life gets when you can't sit or stand. A power wheelchair with zero gravity/reclining function has helped, but the $500 ROHO wheelchair pillow is on top of a flat metal plate, which is incompatible with my adhesive arachnoiditis disability. *Can't Sit: Living with a Sitting Disability* by Rick Lunkenheimer is a valuable firsthand account and reaffirms the sitting problems patients encounter in the outside world, although the author, thankfully, seems to have standing capability. [125]

I felt comfortable going to a movie theater and watching a movie while lying down on the floor, my friend next to me, sitting. To me, lying down was justified because it was my first-year post-accident; my sacrum and lower back still showed a huge, visible swelling. Later, when I was trying to fit back into society, I felt too embarrassed, so I'd bring an inconspicuous stadium seat/bag. Finally, I had to start lying down everywhere, even at open mics at a bar, when I'd bring a camping mat. I survived jobs and academics by spending my lunch hour lying down on an exam table or underneath a desk in a corner. I also missed out on socialization with classmates—never my strongest point, so it was an even more painful experience. But if you've got a sitting disability, or severe pain, you already know that.

Acute Flare-Ups

I obtain a little relief by giving myself weekly Toradol (ketorolac) 60 mg intramuscular injections in the gluteal—buttock—muscle. Ask your provider if he or she can prescribe for home use. Ketorolac is a strong anti-inflammatory and non-opioid pain reliever with a high safety profile, if your labs and kidney function are normal. As noted previously, once or twice a year I also use a short course of steroids called a PredPak.

Dr. Tennant recommends intermittent steroidal use for acute and chronic adhesive arachnoiditis, but I haven't been able to convince my pain team to put me on a continuous, low steroidal dose. Providers seem concerned about bone loss or other side effects, probably rightfully so, but looking at the big picture, my main concern is survival right now. You know, since adhesive arachnoiditis is not compatible with life itself.

Most importantly, re-evaluate what's happening in your life, prioritize, try not to be discouraged. Once you have a little energy, check out the RSDSA website for minimizing flare-ups, or Dr Tennant's strategies.[126] Remember, every patient with neuropathic, or chronic pain will go through bad days and good days and will experience flare-ups, sometimes it helps to vent or post to your Facebook groups.

Environmental Modification

Whenever I venture outside, usually in my power wheelchair, I carry an array of helpful survival tools in my backpack. This includes earplugs; they are bright green, and I cut them in half, so they are a little less conspicuous. The outside world is too noisy for my pained central nervous system, and this includes hearing. Loud music, the bleep bleep of the bus unloading its ramp, cars, people yapping, etc.

I wear earplugs in movie theaters too, as the sound is always loud especially the ads, the coming attractions and explosions. I can only venture outside my studio by protecting myself as much as possible. I carry a light, wool blanket, handy in both winter and in summer—against a nasty, cold air conditioning or swamp cooler system aka evaporative. Carry gloves for bowel care, baby wipes, Hot Toes—found in hunting supply stores or on Amazon to keep your feet warm because cold worsens the pain. Hand sanitizer, sunscreen, and an extra scarf help, as well. Whatever you need to make yourself more comfortable in the environment, do it.

Guilt

Your chronic disease is not your fault; don't waste energy by beating yourself up!

RESOURCES

(All links work as of December 31, 2019)

Better than Oprah's, better than GOOP's shopping guides, and a phenomenal, zero amount of organic, expensive cashmere sweaters: Kaatje's Favorite Things, an Amazon public list with books, practical/stylish home and pain modifications.

Other resources for chronic pain and/or adhesive arachnoiditis, including ketamine providers:

1. American Society of Ketamine Providers A professional, reputable group which hosts yearly conferences since 2018. Reached out to them and haven't heard back. Their website has location info, but not all ketamine clinics are in their directory, which is through a paid membership.
2. Adhesive Arachnoiditis: An Old Disease Re-emerges in Modern Times, by Dr. Tennant, with Ingrid Hollis. Short book that is dedicated to adhesive arachnoiditis, included for free with Kindle Unlimited. Check out his recently published *Handbook to Live Well with Adhesive Arachnoiditis*, it's a great resource for anyone with neuropathic pain, delves into neuroinflammation medications and most importantly, provides hope.
3. Arachnoiditis.co.uk Fantastic website, originally started by Dr. Sarah Smith-Fox as "the A-word" (Dr. Smith-Fox suffers from arachnoiditis herself).
4. Arachnoiditis Hope by Dr. Tennant. Helpful website, PDFs, bulletins for your providers and latest info.
5. The Burton Report by Dr. Burton. Accurate medical website with a lot of history on adhesive arachnoiditis.
6. Face-facts by Red Lawhern, PhD and pain advocate for the Alliance for the Treatment of Intractable Pain. Phenomenal advocacy, research and website for patients, medical providers,

researchers and politicians.

7. <u>Handbook to Live Well with Adhesive Arachnoiditis</u> by Dr. Tennant, with Ingrid Hollis. Thorough companion guide, with the latest treatment on adhesive arachnoiditis. Free with Kindle Lending.

8. <u>Injection & Infusion Clinic</u> Albuquerque, NM. Wonderful clinic treating psychiatric complaints and pain. They provide ketamine troches for at home use in between treatments.

9. <u>Jobri Wedge Pillow Bedrest</u> Instead of a hospital bed, this wedge may be helpful. Listed here as it's available on Google but not Amazon.

10. <u>Ketamine Advocacy Network</u> Could not get confirmed whether that site was actively maintained, blogs date from 2016. To my email I received no reply, though between ASKP, Google and this directory you should be able to find a provider. Don't forget, ask you medical provider or pain team for inpatient infusions and/or oral or intranasal ketamine.

11. <u>Ketamine Infusion Centers</u> Phoenix, AZ and Bakersfield, CA. One of the few centers that will submit billing to your insurance. Like Ketamine Wellness Centers, it is the most reasonably priced, although I have heard of $500 infusions and other clinics actually billing insurance, via FB posts.

12. <u>Ketamine Wellness Centers</u> aka KWC in Mesa, AZ and five other locations in Tucson, CO, TX, MN and WA. The most reasonably priced of all outpatient clinics, with private rooms and flatscreen for YouTube. A Paramedic or Nurse will be in the room with you. KWC has cookies and snacks for after your treatment, tea and coffee. They even kept my post infusion treat, a Diet Rockstar cold. Because you can't eat or drink during a treatment, and a few hours beforehand, your mouth will get dry. KWC provides lemon flavored glycerin swabs during an infusion.

13. <u>Ketamine Research Institute</u> KRIYA You will find a list of medical and mental health providers who specialize in ketamine and ketamine assisted psychotherapy. KRIYA is a professional group with a yearly conference, that seems to use a slightly different approach which emphasizes the *psychospiritual* aspect of ketamine.

14. <u>Minimizing Pain Flare Ups webpage</u> by RSDSA, ways to minimize neuropathic pain, by patients with CRPS—who also describe agonizing, burning pain as part of their syndrome.
15. <u>Practical Pain Management Arachnoiditis Article</u> by **Dr. Tennant.**
16. <u>Practical Pain Management Suspecting Adhesive Arachnoiditis Article</u> by **Dr. Aldrete.**
17. <u>Reflex Sympathetic Dystrophy Syndrome Association</u>'s slogan is "Helping those affected by RSD," it is one of the best resources for neuropathic pain, or any chronic, severe pain disorder. Professional, ethical, compassionate and transparent patient organization with a wealth of research, articles, videos and helpful sources. They have a Treatments page, under Research/Medical, and list a lot of the medications also used for neuropathic pain disorders.

Supportive, resourceful Facebook Groups:

1. <u>Alliance for the Treatment of Intractable Pain</u>
2. <u>Arachniacs: Finding Hope Living with Arachnoiditis</u>
3. <u>Arachnoiditis</u>
4. <u>Arachnoiditis & Chronic Meningitis Collaborative Research Network (ACMCRN)</u>
5. <u>Arachnoiditis and Intractable Pain Advocacy</u>
6. <u>Arachnoiditis Everyday</u>
7. <u>Arachnoiditis from Childbirth Epidural/Spinal Anesthesia</u>
8. <u>Arachnoiditis - Learning to Live Again</u>
9. <u>Arachnoiditis Society</u>
10. <u>Arachnoiditis Society for Awareness and Prevention</u>
11. <u>Arachnoiditis Together We Fight</u>
12. <u>Cauda Equina & Adhesive Arachnoiditis Chronic Disease Pain Neuropathy</u>
13. <u>Chronic Pain Patients News Network</u>
14. <u>Dealing with Arachnoiditis</u>
15. <u>Ket-amine infusions for Better Health</u>
16. <u>Life with Arachnoiditis</u>
17. <u>Tarlov Cyst Society of America</u>

Movies and TV shows that may help prepare your mind a tad, before your first ketamine infusion—there's a lot of sci-fi; to me, every scene in space mimics the ketamine experience. During an infusion, I prefer to watch/listen to gentle relaxation music, meditative YouTube channels, the Mindfulness meditation by Jon Kabatt Zin, or Miriam Makeba to keep me tethered in the here and now. Although I've heard of patients who enjoy watching horror movies while getting a treatment, so whatever you fancy. It's *your* healing journey.

Undone, on Amazon Prime. Episodes 2-5 showcases the infusions' side effects—at some point, the protagonist is in a hospital bed, with civilizations rising and falling in front of her. Inception, Stranger Things, The OA, Black Mirror, The Good Place, Dark, Moon, The Expanse, Melancholia, Spirited Away, Brazil, Memento, Life of Pi, Salaam Bombay, Another Earth, Hair, Russian Doll, Vanity Fair—UK 2018 with fabulous soundtrack, Time Bandits, Princess Mononoke, The Spirits Within, The Expanse, Battlestar Galactica—the remake, and Lost in Space.

ACKNOWLEDGMENTS

Above all lie our motivations for being and belonging, connecting, our core mentality and compassion, our sense of justice and fairness, and our motivation to be healthy and loving. - Greenberg 2010,[127] *Wolfson 2013,*[128] *The Ketamine Papers*

A massive *dank je* and love to my bestie, Nicole van Loon, whose beautiful friendship has endured for over 35 years. Love and a high five to my mom, sis, bro and dad. My deepest gratitude to the medical providers who either literally saved my life, or greatly improved the quality of my life: Jonathan DelosSantos, PA-C, Chera, Mandeep and the supportive, welcoming team at the Ketamine Wellness Center in Mesa, AZ; CNP Katherine Devine's helpful Infusion and Injections Clinic in Albuquerque; cheerleader and therapist Hope Varela; Physical Therapist, and custom insoles genius Bone Dexter; my dedicated, smart primary care provider and terrific friend, Cynthia Weir, CFNP; and to our family's fantastische primary care physician Dr. Moekti in Holland.

To the Rio Grande Hospital Pain Management Team, Dr Rogelj, Dr Sol and medical staff, nursing team, medical assistants, and clerks: what an amazing, healing journey it's been. Thanks to you, I have hope. And since there aren't enough words to fit on a Thank You card, I wrote a book. And thank *you*, Professor Calvin Stevens. You synthesized ketamine in 1962, and wow, did you do the world a favor. Your contribution to humanity's wellbeing cannot be underestimated, on par with Norman Borlaug's Green Revolution. Better living through chemistry, indeed.

Special shout out to Forest Tennant, M.D., Dr.PH, for his unwavering support of patients with adhesive arachnoiditis. Dr. Tennant's Practical Pain Management contributions, and his practical bulletins geared to patients and their providers are an ongoing source of superior knowledge, and hope.

Another special shout out to Red Lawhern, PhD and advocate, founder of the Alliance for the Treatment of Intractable Pain—ATIP—bringing together advocates, scientists, patients and medical providers. Every day, Dr. Lawhern fights for the human right to be treated for chronic, severe pain, a right which has steadily eroded these past few years.

A heartfelt thanks to the unsung heroes of the medical field: The Rapid Response Team for my IVs; the PICC Team for my midline IVs; the kind janitors; the caring and hardworking Techs. Kayla Crites; kudos for finding my retainers, you saved the day. Hardworking power wheelchair technicians Chris and Joshua from Numotion, for keeping Ms. Hot Wheels on the road, and a big high five to Numotion wheelchair tech Angel, who solved a three-and-a-half-year power wheelchair problem.

George Sikkink and the stellar team at Downtown New Mexico Sports & Wellness, for keeping my mind and body happy; there is no other way I would have made it this far. Athlete and trainer Meredith 'Merf' Hardy and fellow gym member Carla, thank you so much for proofreading, morale-boosting and the exercise classes. Albuquerque City Drug: Pete Sedillo, Pharm.D, and staff for your compassion, home delivery and meeting me at my car for a flu vaccine or meds.

Olive Tree Compounding Pharmacy's Ndidiamaka 'Didi' Okpareke, Pharm.D for your expertise, kindness and care, preparing and mailing ketamine troches. Ivy Rose Gonzales, *the* New Mexico seating specialist, Compassus Home Health Occupational and Physical Therapists, RNs and Medical Social Worker for the TLC, to this day I faithfully perform your PT & OT exercises.

Cindi Allen, Raphaela Francis, PA-C, Jamie Bailon, PA-C, Laura Johnson, CNP and Alejandro Lopez: thank you for bringing friendship, food and uplifting feedback into my life when I really needed it. To Kim DeLauter-Taylor, Debbie Grady M.D., Claude Langlois, Celeste 'Spoken' Garcia, David Garcia, Danny Danger, Chris Nakai, Julie and Margaret Farrer, Carol Hjellming, Megan Heisenberg Harmeyer, Laura Loeber Foreman, Barbara Lemaire, Dr. Blue, Adam James, and others for your uplifting friendship.

Much gratitude to Nash Jones, Jamie Campbell and Marty Adam Smith for lighting the fire of comedy and storytelling. Curt Fletcher and Kris Shaw for The Crippled Comedy Tour and most of all, for your friendship and encouragement. Edward McDonald, Brigitte van Beek-Wagemakers, Brigitta van der Linden, Gillian Gaggero-Gazollo, Peter Bjerg and Anne Marie Hoogeveen: love you and miss you.

Muchas gracias, friends and neighbors Terri Krantz and precious little Pearl, Mike Long, Erick Dang, Janelle Gutierrez, Kay Mason, Mark Price,

Terry Graff and Rusty Rutherford for kindness, pushing my manual wheelchair, pharmacy errands, taking me to the gun range and picking me up from the hospital. A very special thank you to Dylan Tsosie, an extraordinarily Navajo oil painter and friend, for having faith in me and my comedy, from the moment we met.

Christy Cutter for the excellent editing and support, Grammar Girl for succinct teaching 24/7; Jared Anaya, muchas gracias for your friendship and fixing my laptop, which enabled me to finish this manuscript. Dear Audrey McNamara, Ursula van den Hurk Voets, Alan Morris, Andrew van Etten, Jennifer DeSantis, Astrid van den Worm, Laura Loeber Foreman, Chase Martin, comic Jesse Ever and all other off- and online friends; thanks for your support. Sonia, Ray, Antonio and Sam from Ray's Smoke Shop; thanks for your friendliness, coconut ice cream and Diet Dr Pepper so I could finish this book.

My sweet friends from Hoensbroek Spinal Cord Injury Rehabilitation Hospital: John Geven, Raf Linmans, Rico Ramdhan and Frans Meulbroek. After all these years, you remain a guiding light in my life, which now includes the lovely and talented Nicole van der Maazen—John's wife. Francisco Soto, very grateful for your attitude, friendship and morale boosting, homie. My old skydiving friends Jan, Arij, Monique, Ralph and Charlie Orchard; blue skies, dear ones.

My fellow arachniacs Lori Verton, Donna Corley, Kris Walters—meeting you was the highlight of the Crippled Comedy Tour, Marlisa Griffith, Carol Palackdharry M.D., Allison Tucker, Robert West, Mara Downes McGrail— your TLC packages with icepacks are the bomb, Arlene Lawson, Scott Groves, Casey Muse Bendig, Dawn Gonzalez, Brad Franklin, Kelly Jo, Sherri Freezman, Louise Carbonneau, Joanne Spevack, Teresa Haney, Rhonda Posey, Tiina Säynäjoki, Deirdre Kitchen, Shauncey Maver, Dawn M. Rasjl Barajas, Janet Finley and others: let's keep fighting the good fight.

Matthew McDuffy, this memoir wouldn't have been the same without your stellar lecture on The Hero's Journey and storytelling. I was scared to share this 'elixir' with the world, until I realized that everything you discussed was already in the memoir, such as *Gravity*, fractals and Aristotle. Basil Hoffman and Brad Lemack: much gratitude for pointing me towards the light. Atlanta DJ Many for cheering me up during a rough patch, offering to fly in and sleep with me. You're A1. Taos classmates Brian Wolfe and Mishele Maron; thanks so much for your feedback and pep talk.

Perhaps the single greatest contributor to this book is South-African singer and human rights activist Miriam Makeba, aka Mama Africa. Whenever I couldn't write, edit or research from pain and exhaustion, Miriam's music and spirit emboldened me to keep going. John Callahan's cartoons and memoir have inspired me for over 25 years, and so has the music of Curtis Mayfield, whose accident during a 1993 Brooklyn concert left him with quadriplegia. John Restivo and Bill 'Bad Spot' van Texel: you witnessed my fall from a few feet away and saw me bounce, then willed me to live. There are no words.

P.S.

In the end, ketamine is many things to many people, but most of all it is hope.
- Stephen J. Hyde, MD, The Ketamine Papers [129]

Dear reader, despite the hard work, and worsening pain that *The Queen of Ketamine* required, I am grateful. I learned much more than anticipated, and strongly feel as though we took this pilgrimage together. With a chronic illness and/or disability, it's almost easier to operate in survival mode, especially looking at a long to-do list with a body, or mind, that doesn't cooperate. After years of struggling, that kind of thinking feels familiar, right? Yet, I would like for you—and I—to create spare energy. That way you can finally enjoy a hobby, connect with—an online—community, and learn to experience joy again. You deserve joy.

Most chronic diseases, including mental health disorders, are cyclical, so there are days you will feel better than others. My sister Nicolien taught me that in an Eindhoven brewpub when she was in Nursing school, although it would take two decades before I understood her wise words. You may experience weeks, months or years of improvement, or regretfully, decline. Be patient with yourself. When you do feel good, or *better*, try to save some energy for happiness *and* for unexpected situations, e.g., an acute illness, bad news, an exhausting day at work or a doctor's appointment that takes twice as long. You deserve a better quality of life, so let's make it happen.

Because of the severity of the pain disorder, I was prescribed a hospital bed after the 2015 hospitalization. It has an electric foot and headrest adjustments. A friend gave me a memory foam mattress and for me, it's the most comfortable way to live. Before the hospital bed, I used the more labor-intensive wedges and footrests, as described in Resources. I have mostly left out the term *central sensitization* and will address that in my second memoir, *The Queen of Kratom.* Hold your horses, it's just a catchy title, I won't be recommending kratom. Probably.

The second memoir contains events from October 2017 through

December 2019; eight weeklong hospital ketamine infusions, more outpatient infusions, criminal summons, a splendid but ill-fated TEDx talk, finances, hosting The Crippled Comedy Tour, and a gnarly rear-ending. While performing a final fact check before publication, it would be disingenuous to withhold that out of desperation, the last two months I've been on a strict anti-inflammatory diet.

I even added Dr. Tennant's recommended daily supplements—pregnenolone, DHEA, colostrum—and fish oil capsules my best friend raved about. Through Amazon and a zero-interest credit card, I bought an Ootori SL track massage chair, and I started working out harder and stretching deeper. My efforts seem to make an enormous difference in my wellbeing. Most importantly, I live to fight another day, for another book. Thanks *so* much for sticking around, see you at *The Queen of Kratom*.

Love, Kaatje

PS: If you've enjoyed this book, leave a review on Amazon.com. I would also appreciate feedback if links no longer work or if you find an error, no matter how small. Please contact me via email, or via my website. Follow me on Facebook for updates.

THE ULTIMATE MIRIAM MAKEBA PLAYLIST

Throughout the years this book required, I only listened to Miriam Makeba, via records or YouTube. These one-hour collections on YouTube deserve a mention, as they're usually played without ads: *Uganda Radio Makeba Music* and *Mama Africa Origins Full Albums*. Here is an overview of my favorite records and songs. Enjoy!

"Miriam Makeba" RCA 1960, produced by Harry Belafonte

- Where does it lead
- Nomeva (Xosa love song, sung during weddings)
- The Click Song (festive Xosa song)
- Umhume (Swasi lament, about being betrayed by a friend)
- Mbube (Zulu song about a lion hunt)

On the back of the LP Harry Belafonte writes: "Sparks were there in Miss Makeba's artistry and her strangely powerful songs. Knowing her and working with Miriam Makeba counts as one of my greatest artistic privileges."

"The Magnificent Miriam Makeba" Mercury Records 1966, produced by Luchi de Jesus

- Mr Man
- La Bushe (Congo bushe)
- Charlie (Oh mama)
- That's how it goes (Ntsizwa)
- Oh tell me my mother

Luchi de Jesus writes: "I deem it a high point in my career to have had the opportunity to add my own creative efforts to her insurmountable ones."

"Pata Pata" Warner Brothers 1967, arranged and produced by Luchi de Jesus

- Ring bell, ring bell
- Westwind
- A piece of ground
- What is love (a crafty, melancholic arrangement with violins!)
- Maria Fulo

Hal Halverstadt writes, most likely when he had just smoked a big spliff, although his seemingly over the top blurb *is* the truth: "Miss Makeba. A trip to the moon on brightly feathered wings. The sweetest nose cone this side of Heaven. And the most exciting space age phenomena since Telstar." Arranged and produced by Luchi de Jesus, who writes: "Second outing with Reprise Records (the first, 'Miriam Makeba in Concert'!)."

Fav songs not owned on records but via YouTube:

- L'Enfant et la Gazelle
- We got to make it
- Lumumba
- Soweto Blues (written by Hugh Masekela)
- I'mm You'mm We'mm
- Mas Que Nada
- Oxgam
- Lindelani
- Dubula
- Love tastes like strawberries
- Malaika
- Congo

I've listened to Miriam since before I was born; my father played her records and her South-African lullabies when my mom was pregnant. It's the sound of my childhood, and now such a source of comfort. In 2017 I started buying her records after finding her songs on YouTube. A small old-fashioned looking record player was only $31 on-line, and her records are cheap, some are $1.98 on Discogs.com. One of my records came from Detroit, from the first owner in 1962. How neat is that?

At age 20 I dated this vain artist/model from Afghanistan. We lived in a cold loft above his uncle's fast food chicken restaurant in Williamsburg, the second subway stop from the bridge. Such a jerk, he didn't plan anything for my 20th birthday. And so, I went to Carnegie Hall alone, where Miriam Makeba, aka Mama Africa, gave a sold-out concert with Hugh Masekela. Her audience knew what it meant to see this legend and that Miriam Makeba wasn't granted permission (from the South-African government) to attend her mother's funeral. She had been banned from her country for 31 years.

After the skydiving accident, I worked on a ship called the Stella Maris, as sailor and server for the upscale clientele. A ship was actually good for me; limited walking, using ladders, not having to cook, and I loved the maintenance. The greatest difficulty of course, was jumping from the ship to shore and my left leg greatly suffered. We were moored in Amsterdam for a few weeks, behind the red-light district and I attended Miriam's concert in a nightclub. It was a bit pitiful, such a small gig, just before "World Music" would get hip again through Putamayo records. It seemed that Mama Africa, one of the best and most creative voices of her generation, had fallen on hard times, with bad managers.

In the mid-nineties we saw Miriam Makeba as a family, with my parents, sister and brother. What a great memory, of a World Music festival in Rotterdam, with her granddaughter singing and dancing. I could not stand on my legs for long and managed to put a chair all the way in front. I like to think that Miriam Makeba must not have minded the ebbs and flows of her career. She was unapologetically herself, whether in Carnegie Hall or a shitty Amsterdam night club, it did not matter. That's how great she was.

To recall the physical reality of the African continent—and that of all developing nations and much of humanity before industrialization and the Green Revolution—one of her songs, Ngola Kurila, is simple described as: "A woman pacifies her hungry child. There is nothing to eat." (There's good news too; the last 30 years a billion people were lifted out of poverty.) Miss Makeba did what she could to propel beauty, endurance and hope forward, and we are blessed with her legacy. The magnificent Miriam Makeba passed away shortly after performing at an Italian jazz festival.